the Ruby Rose Hotel, Etta's and the Billionaires

Garth Lewis

Acknowledgments

While writing this book two of my greatest and dearest friends passed away. This book is dedicated to Bob Paffile and Jim Eisele. Grade school, high school, college, the army, and many beers beyond, rest in peace my friends.

I would like to thank Etta for all the kindness and gracefulness she has bestowed upon me throughout the lifetime of our friendship. If it had not been for Etta this book would not been written and we would have never shared the pleasure and joy of reading it.

I would like to say thank you to my friend Richard Hines. Rich volunteered his time and expertise knowledge in cleaning up my English.

Damon Glatz, my publishing expert, who put up with me with very little financial rewards, thank you Damon. And thank all the wonderful people at BookBaby.

Morgan, on the 310 to Yuma, thanks.

Introduction

All my life I have been into sports, baseball, football, basketball, golf, tennis, swimming and a few others. I was not a good athlete, not big, not strong or fast, but I enjoyed the game. I graduated from college with a Bachelors of Arts Degree in Radio Broadcasting with the intent on becoming a sports broadcaster. After a few years in the broadcasting business it didn't go well for me so I left the trade and became a carpenter. I found this more to my liking, it was the physical movement I enjoyed, the sweat, the good energy well spent, and the concentration, that motivated me.

When I retired from carpentry I went back to college and received my certification to become a personal fitness trainer. I have combined my broadcasting experience with my fitness experience to pen this book.

The Ruby Rose Hotel, Etta's and the Billionaires is a health and fitness novel directed to the hundreds of guys and gals, young and old, who spend hours and hours each day in fitness clubs across the land improving their lives. The grind, the commitment, the effort to keep improving is what keeps these people going. This book is for them.

To make the book a tad more interesting and fun to read I have added a caper to the story, the robbery at the Ruby Rose Hotel. This is the first of four novel featuring Johnny Tucson, GeeGee Gambino, Carman Fish, Stella and a few others.

All the questions asked of Johnny, and GeeGee on the radio talk show, "Fitness for the Day," are authentic questions asked of me during my years of training.

In between the phone calls Carman Fish has mustered up a gang of thieves to rob the Ruby Rose Hotel the night of the Billionaires Gala. Carman's crew consists of hard working honest Americans citizens who have come up on the short end of the dollar. But they hang in there, believing in the old axiom, hard work and honest living pays off.

By all means, if you plan on exercising please consult with your care giver first.

DO NOT, UNDER ANY CIRCUMSTANCES use any exercise in this book without consulting a fitness trainer they are for this book only.

THE RUBY ROSE HOTEL, ETTA'S, AND THE BILLIONAIRES

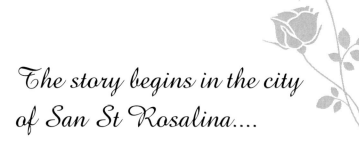

The story begins in the city of San St Rosalina....

The fog is lifting and the seagulls are squawking as the sun breaks the horizon and begins a slow rise over the city.

It is early morning in the southwest corner of America, the tide is low, and the smell of the Pacific Ocean filters through the early morning mist, signaling the beginning of a new day; bacon and eggs are on, potatoes and onions are frying, and coffee is up.

Johnny Tucson powers the old wooden boat down, and slowly motors past the jetty and carefully maneuvers through the opening that separates the jetty from the spit. The tramper nudges its nose into the marina and travels at a snail's pace, ever so careful as not to leave a wake.

As it motors gently and quietly past the workboats and beyond the pleasure craft, the big boat stays the course, slow and steady until it comes to the slip it will call home, 903, D Dock, Sunset Bay Marina.

Johnny finishes securing the last of the mooring lines, hoists his duffel bag up onto his shoulder and makes his way up the steep gangway, out of the marina basin and onto the city streets.

Johnny stands tall, pumps his fists, stretches his arms and legs, and embraces the good feeling of standing on solid bedrock after five days on the rolling ocean.

He walks across the parking lot that separates the marina from the spit; he steps onto the flagstone walkway leading to Etta's Restaurant. Johnny walks past the Polish hot dog stand, the flower, vegetable, and herb gardens, moves under the arbors and keep on walking until he enters the front door of Etta's for a well-deserved beer and breakfast.

Johnny had just motored eleven hundred miles down the Pacific Ocean from Portland, Oregon, to San St. Rosalina. The sky was gray, the sea was angry, and the tramper was rolling and pitching all the way; Johnny deserves more than a beer and breakfast, but what the hell!

Etta's is a hand-me-down restaurant. Etta's great-great-grandfather started the business by selling shrimp from his boat, which he moored to that same jetty well over a hundred years ago. The business was handed down, hand over hand, through the family chain and stayed much the same until Etta's father, Tony, took over. Tony, with city approval, erected a forty-foot tent on the spit from which he not only sold shrimp, but he also sold herring, smelt, and tuna, as well as tomatoes, onions, and peppers.

The business became so good for Tony he bought the spit from the city and constructed a post and beam open-air building. To this he added and added, when Etta took over the business she added and added, changed the name from Tony's to Etta's and it is what it is.

"Good morning, and welcome to "Fitness for the Day. I'm GeeGee Gambino filling in for Johnny Tucson.

"And what a lovely morning it is, cool and crispy, blue sky and a yellow sun rising; the leaves on the trees are gold and orange with a tint of red and a smidgen of green; oh, this just tickles my heart, I love it!"

"We have Shirley on the line, Shirley, how can I help you?"

"GeeGee, good morning, and thank you for taking my call, I'm a first-time caller but a long-time listener. I've been listening to Johnny Tucson for years, I hope he enjoys his new boat, when will he be back?"

"He's southbound from Portland as we speak, should be in town any day. What can I help you with today, Shirley?"

"GeeGee, I've been trying to lose weight for years, but all I seem to do is gain. I've tried this diet that diet, listened to my friend Anne, who is as skinny as a rail. I've joined several fitness clubs, talked with doctors, talked to other friends, to this person that person, all have advised me, but nothing works. It seems so hopeless, GeeGee, I'm only forty-seven years old, what can I do?"

"One thing for sure, Shirley, you're not a quitter you never give up, and above all else that's what it takes to lose weight, never give up."

"You're right about that, GeeGee. I keep trying, plugging away, probably will be doing so until the day I die."

"Shirley, there are many so-called, 'Weight Loss Resorts,' throughout the country, have you tried any of them?

"Well, no I haven't, I don't even know what,' Weight Loss Resorts,' are."

"They're similar to alcoholic treatment centers only these resorts are for people who desperately want to lose weight. You go there for one, two, maybe three months; you stay there twenty-four hours a day, seven days a week. You eat from their menu, do their exercise programs, and follow their advice. When you leave, they say, 'good-bye, Rail,' because you're as skinny as a rail, just like your friend Anne."

"You do follow-ups every year or so to keep you in check. They keep you coming back, you keep the pounds off." "Plus, Shirley, they are resorts, so you swim, hot tub, sauna, bike ride, and all kinds of wonderful activities. And the big plus here is they are filled with people in the same boat as you, so it's easy to make friends, socialize and have fun."

"These places do work, Shirley, people have been known to drop a hundred or so pounds at these resorts."

"I wonder how expensive they are?"

"Look into it; maybe you're talking two, three, four thousand dollars a month, depending on which resort you choose and what package you buy."

"Shirley, there are several other less expensive private organizations like Jenny Craig, Weight Watchers, and Nutrisystem. There are also many public organizations like Over-eaters Anonymous and Lose Pounds Sensibility that are free, have you tried any of these places?"

"Well, no again."

"More places to check out, but I'll tell you what I recommend; I recommend you hire a personal fitness trainer. Have you ever hired a personal fitness trainer, Shirley?"

"No I haven't, I guess I have more options open to me than I thought."

"Spend some money and do the job right, Shirley. Doctors are Doctors and friends are friends, but fitness trainers will get you down the road of slim and narrow." "They get in the grind with you not just advise you! They're on the mat with you, they're on the bench with you, and they're beside you all the way, coaching, teaching, and listening. They work hand in hand with you, Shirley!"

And when you're not in the gym the trainer keeps pushing you on proper nutrition, without proper nutrition everything goes to hell in a hand basket. And accountability, remember accountability from grade school and high school, you had to be accountable to the teacher, same thing here, if you do not achieve your fitness goals the trainer will let you know."

"Personal trainers are the real deal, honey; hire one, and I guarantee you'll become the New You!"

"Tell you what; I'm penciling this conversation on my board as we speak. I would like you to call me back, let's see, today is December sixth, call me back the first week in February and tell me what's happening."

"Now you have accountability, Shirley, you're accountable to me, you're accountable to the listening audience, and you will be accountable to your personal trainer. Let's get this job rolling sweetheart; we want to hear good things from you. And remember, **there is no finish line, Shirley, it's a lifetime commitment.**"

"Wonderful, GeeGee! This sounds great, just great, I'm excited, I really am! This is going to be fun, money well spent, and I'm looking forward to it."

"Tomorrow, I'll get with a personal trainer and the new Shirley will be calling you back in February. Thank you so much, GeeGee."

"Adios Shirley, we'll talk soon."

"Say, friends, if you are trying to lose weight, Etta's Restaurant, at Sunset Bay Marina, is the perfect place to begin. Etta's offers the Daily Meal Plan; you can have breakfast hot off the stove, eggs, garden fresh potatoes, toast and jam, only five hundred calories and it tastes like home cooking." "How about lunch in a bag, a tuna sandwich mixed with avocado, tomatoes and a sprinkle of Tabasco, only three hundred and ninety calories!"

"All this along with a big juicy orange plucked fresh off the tree."

"Etta's counts the calories for you. You feel good all day without that bloated feeling and you'll lose weight and gain energy. Why not buy the ninety-day meal plan and see how good you feel at the end of three months?"

"Just call or stop by Etta's and talk the talk with the people who talk the talk of health and nutrition."

"Hi, you're on Fitness for the Day, with GeeGee Gambino. How can I help you?"

"Hi, GeeGee, my name is Roy and I'm calling from Ocean Bay. I just wanted to tell the previous caller I did the same thing she did and nothing worked for me either. Weeks and weeks went by, I talked to this person, that person, try this try that, nothing was working. Finally one day I said to myself, 'the hell with all this, I'm hiring a trainer!"

"It was the smartest move I ever made. I began losing weight, my arms and legs became stronger, my core began to harden, and I was energized! This was right out of the gate, I was amazed!"

"Cardio was brought into play, stretching was introduced, and nutrition was added. The learning never stops, GeeGee, I learned how important is to keep a log book, how to use the equipment properly, and how to chart the foods I eat, good-bye cheesy this and creamy that and hello fruits and veggies!"

"I've lost forty-seven pounds, added muscle, and changed my body composition: my body fat went from a whopping thirty-three percent to a respectable twenty-one percent, I feel wonderful, GeeGee; I recommend hiring a trainer from the get-go!"

"It's been two years, and I'm still going strong and still with the same trainer, plus, I've brought in two friends, it's been great" "I just wanted to tell Shirley this, GeeGee, thanks for taking my call."

"Good-bye, Roy, wonderful story, keep up the good work and thank you for calling."

"Shirley, I hope you had your radio on and your ears tuned in, get a trainer and a workout partner, **keep it smart.**"

The old wooden tramper is moored about two hundred yards down the marina shoreline from Etta's. She's a 1966 Swedish motor sailor made of Teak planks, Oak, and Mahogany wood. The boat is seventy feet long at the waterline and twenty-eight feet wide amidships. She is powered by a newly refitted Detroit Diesel engine and two masks of sails; in nautical language she is called a Yawl. In her working days she sailed up and down the Pacific Coast from Astoria, Oregon to Seattle, Washington. She hauled frozen shrimp, fish, and crab on her way up and on the return trip, she dropped off potatoes, peas, corn, and wheat at the same docks. Johnny plans on refurbishing the old gal and taking her on a world cruise. However, first thing first, he has the boat, now he needs a crew.

Etta's is flanked on the north by Sunset Bay Marina, on the west by the Pacific Ocean, on the east by the city of San St. Rosalina, and on the south by the Ruby Rose Hotel.

The Ruby Rose Hotel is a 114-room state-of-the-art horseshoe-shaped four-story stucco building. It offers valet parking, a courtyard, scenic views for all guests, and a shopping mall.

The subfloor of the hotel plays host to the fashionable mall. Shoppers will find clothing stores for men, women, and children, dozens of outstanding boutiques, beauty shops, barbershops, banks, specialty stores, business offices, racquetball courts, bowling lanes, and The Cobbler Shop.

The ground floor is the gateway to the hotel, opening into a beautiful full-service lobby to include car rentals, airline agents, bagel and coffee shops, floral stores, and two excellent restaurants, The Shamrock Room and the Kingfisher. There are movie theaters, sweet shops, The Pizzeria, The Hamburger Joint, many import stores, and several specially promoted hotel suites.

The second and third floors of the hotel offer 114 spacious three-room suits, featuring king-size beds, 48-inch plasma TV's, walk-in showers, kitchenettes, and decks with Jacuzzi. The guests on the west side of the hotel have an unimpeded view of all ships and pleasure craft moving in and about Sunset Bay. Every evening there is a show of splendor and a soft splash of pastel color as the sun sets on the horizon. Guests on the east side of the hotel have a wonderful evening view of San St. Rosalina's city cape as well as a dynamic sunrise.

Rooms located on the inside of the horseshoe offer views of the courtyard. Three acres of green grass, shade trees, orange trees, hedges, flower gardens, and a forty by the twenty-five-foot kidney-shaped swimming pool with a swim-up bar. Guests also find themselves with a lovely view of Sunset Bay Marina.

The fourth floor of the Ruby Rose is for meetings, a dance studio, a stretching studio, several art studios, six executive offices, and a home for the hotel owners, Greg and Kelly Diamond. The large banquet room, where the Billionaires Gala Invitational is held, is also on the fourth floor. `

Cameron Blue has operated the main elevator of the Ruby Rose Hotel for five years. Cameron has an MBA in Business Finance and had been working as a comptroller at an engineering firm. At age thirty-six, with death staring him in the face, Cameron made a career switch to a simpler way of life.

DH Jimmy owns and operates The Cobbler Shop, where he has been making, mending, repairing, and shining shoes since the grand opening of the mall six years ago. DH Jimmy and Cameron Blue were high school buddies.

Charmain Green is a blond-haired green-eyed gal from Iowa. She has that down-home look of, 'who me,' as mischief isn't a part of her daily bread. Charmain has been serving drinks in the Captain's Quarters of the Kingfisher Restaurant for sixteen weeks; the clientele is friendly and wealthy.

Charmain is a newbie in town and uses her smile, friendly attitude, and good work ethics to generate handsome tip money.

Carman Fish was a successful offshore drug runner from Miami. He owned a fifty-four-foot "cigarette boat" and for three years managed to outrun and stay one step ahead of the law, but times were changing. The Feds, State, and local authorities, with new and improved equipment were now faster and more efficient both on land and at sea, and were rapidly closing the doors on drug smugglers in the Gulf.

Carman was only twenty-nine years old and did not want to spend time in prison. Although the timing wasn't right Carman made a sudden retirement from his drug running career, sold his boat, packed his belonging, and headed west across the continent.

Carman landed in San St. Rosalina where he has been tending bar in the Shamrock Room for eighteen months. Carman has a plan!

"Roll over Beethoven," who wrote that song? Third-person to call in wins a free lunch, courtesy of Etta's.

"Hi, you're on Fitness for the Day, with Johnny Tucson."

"Hi Johnny, my name is Mike, and I live in Quiet Cove. Welcome back, good to hear your voice again, and congratulations on buying a new boat.

"Thank you, Mike, the boat is not new, just new to me. In fact, she is over fifty years old, and I have plenty of work to do." "Are you a shipwright, Mike?"

"No, I wish I were I would love to help you, bet it would be fun, working on an old boat down on the water."

"I'm not sure about fun, Mike, we'll see. What can I help you with this morning?"

"Johnny, I'm at the gym five days a week and the pointers you throw out are very helpful, but let me ask you this. Everyone is talking about protein smoothies, I would like to know if protein supplements really help, or is that just a physiological ploy to make people think they are doing themselves a big favor by taking additional protein?"

"Mike, if you're at the gym five days a week, lifting, doing cardio, taking a class or two, I would say a teaspoon of protein powder would do you good. Protein is the building block of life; it repairs and rebuilds damaged muscles. If you're doing the heavy lifting, breaking your muscles down every day or so, you need something to help rebuild them, and that's where protein comes in. Drink plenty of water, keep flushing."

"Tell you what, Mike; the best thing to do is talk with a nutritionist. You'll be getting first hand, accurate information. Nutritionists are more into the chemical and science part of the body, whereas I'm into the physical and mechanical aspects of the body. It doesn't hurt to take a different route on this question, a second opinion so to speak."

"Go for a nutritionist on this one, Mike." "Thanks for calling and give me a call back and let me know what is said."

"Ok, Johnny, will do, thanks for taking my call and good luck on the boat."

"The human body is chemistry, anytime a person is going to take supplements on the daily basis it's best to talk with a nutritionist beforehand. Organs in the body run a clean and smooth operation; if they get saturated with too much, 'over the counter goodies,' bad things can happen. The problems may not arise today, but two, three, five years down the road something might surface, so check it out, and be careful."

"We have a winner!" "Gracie from down on Pike Street correctly identified Chuck Berry as the writer of "Roll over Beethoven." Come on down Gracie, and we'll give you a coupon for a free lunch at Etta's."

The "Big Board" at Sunset Bay Marina is an excellent place to pin an ad if you're looking for seafarers. The board is six feet by four feet and is centrally located so all passersby will notice it. If you're looking for a shipwright, welder, laminators, cooks, stewards, captains, or able-bodied mariners, the board is the place to look. Johnny Tucson's ad read as follows:

Looking for an able-bodied mariner, offer free room and board plus a small wage. Must be clean and neat, willing to work twenty-five hours a week. A year's worth of work, a world cruise to follow. D dock; slip 903, Sunset Bay Marina, or ask along the docks for Johnny Tucson.'

Etta looks like the girl next door, young-looking, petit, pretty in the face, thin bones, long black and silver hair, and a flair for the dress. What sets Etta apart from other successful businesswomen is vision; Etta has vision beyond imagination.

A person can go into Etta's Restaurant and dance to live music or catch a DJ spinning records seven days a week; the sailors keep coming, the locals keep dining, the music never stops. Two, three, four o'clock in the morning, a soul can sit, listen, dance, eat, drink, play darts, or shoot pool. It's all there twenty-four hours a day, seven days a week, the restaurant knows no time.

Men wearing thousand-dollar suits can be seen shooting pool with guys wearing baseball caps and fishing boots. There are pinball machines, shuffleboard tables, and three hundred seats for breakfast, lunch, and dinner diners.

Added to the mix are fresh seafood vendors, vegetable vendors, and Italian, Mexican, and Chinese fresh food vendor. There are a dozen plasma TV screens throughout the restaurant and yet there is still plenty of space for those wanting peace and quiet, books and magazines are plentiful.

Etta's is half the size as a football field, with no interior walls and no exterior walls; post and beam construction, with mosquito netting draping the outside.

Etta's father, Tony, in his wildest dreams, had no idea that someday there would be a 14-acre park leading to the entrance of the restaurant. The park includes a half-acre herb garden where diners can pick herbs for their evening meal. Nor did Tony imagine two acres of flowers and vegetable gardens with pathways through these gardens where diners can walk and pick lovely looking and fresh smelling flowers for their dinner table. No, Tony never had that kind of vision, but he was thinking about security though, his model was, "No Drunks, No Fights, No Police, It's Bad for Business." This original sign still hangs at the entrance to the restaurant.

There are plenty of handsome young muscle beach type men and women wearing red, white, and blue button-down shirts with ETTA'S neatly stitched across the front roaming the premises, reason enough for no one to cause trouble.

Tony's wife was Polish so Tony dreamed of a Polish Sausage Vending Cart. Today a cart stands at the entrance of the park, with four tables, benches, shade trees, a drinking fountain, and an arbor. This is where Johnny Tucson was sitting when Stella walked up.

"Hi, are you Johnny Tucson?"

"Yes, I am," Johnny answered, as he looked up and was somewhat taken aback as he eyed the woman standing before him. She had a deep dark tan; stood about five feet ten inches tall, long dark red hair, pale pink lipstick, tattoos on both arms, and a pack of cigarettes rolled up her sleeve. When she removed her sunglasses, her eyes were robin egg blue.

"Hello You," Johnny quietly uttered to himself.

"I asked around the docks, and all fingers pointed to the gentleman sitting next to the Polish Sausage Cart." "My name is Stella; I read your ad on the board concerning an able-bodied mariner." Stella extends her hand in greetings.

Now Johnny enjoys a Polish Sausage more than anyone, but this one had to wait. He pushes his Polish aside, wiped his mouth and hands with the paper napkin, stands and extended his hand to meet Stella's.

In the days leading up to the purchase of the tramper, Johnny had the boat lifted out of the water, dry docked and surveyed; he wanted to know the condition of the boat under the waterline. Was the prop in good shape, was the shaft straight true and sealed, and what did the rudder look like? Was the bottom paint good clean and well cared for or was it peeling and filled with barnacles, was there dry rot in the wood? The bilge was pumped, cleaned, and inspected.

Johnny knew the condition of the boat under the waterline before he purchased it. There would be no surprises and large sums of money to be paid out down the road.

There are plenty of sailors hanging around San St. Rosalina, and there are an equal number of guys and gals pretending to be sailors. The pretenders are looking to climb aboard for a ride to unknown ports in the far-off world while leaving their troubles behind. Much like he needed to know what was under the waterline of the tramper, Johnny needed to know what was under the skin of these sailors, some are true sailors, while others are the pretenders; Johnny needed to know who was who, he used the look, feel, and listen method.

Johnny looks into the face of the prospective hire; is the face time reddened and weathered. Are the lines deep, hardened, and showing experience in the sun, wind, and rain, or is it a face from the office, clean clear and fresh with no hard time and very few signs in the elements.

He looks into the eyes; they are the gateway to the soul. Are the eyes alive, keen, healthy, alert, and ready for action, or are they bloodshot, tired, gray, and decaying from an unhealthy lifestyle?

Are the hands, arms, and legs strong, firm, and steady? Is the handshake the grasp of a working hand, or is it a grip of a pencil pusher? Does the walk have the spring of a light foot, or is it the thud of a lead foot, is the voice strong, clear, and concise?

Johnny needs to know these people; three hundred and sixty-five days at sea is a long time, he better be with the right group? The look, feel, and listen method will tell him plenty, and then it was on to "walk the walk."

Please understand, this is not your typical interview with a resume and cover letter in hand, fancy clothes, polished shoes, and gleaming teeth, no, this is 'come as you are, sit and chat.

Johnny and Stella shake hands.

"Have a seat, Stella; would you care for a Polish, coffee or a soda," Johnny asked, as he gestures with his hand towards his half-eaten lunch?

"No thank you, I had a late breakfast; maybe I'll just get a cup with ice and fill it with water from the fountain." Stella excused herself and returned a few moments later with her drink.

"So, you're an able-bodied mariner."

"Yes, I graduated from Amherst with a master's degree in Marine Biology. From there I hitched a ride on a freighter to France. I had some connections, and it took a while, but finally I was lucky enough to land a job with Jacque Cousteau."

"After seven years of sailing the seas doing oceanography work I returned to the states where I went to work for Shell Oil on an off-shore rig in the Gulf. I did this for two years, and then I went to work as a naturalist on a tour boat."

"Sounds interesting, and today you're looking for a part-time job as an able-bodied mariner."

"Yes, everyone on board a Cousteau boat is an able-bodied mariner, along with the job you were hired for. You're at sea for long periods of time, and there is plenty of boat maintenance to do, scraping, painting, cleaning are part of the gig, everyone chips in. On the oil rig, there was none of that, but on the tour boat it was hands-on every day, I have plenty of experience."

"I've been off work for a couple of years now and would like to get back out on the blue waters. But not necessary as an employee, something a little more fun, with a little more excitement, and adventure! A world cruise sounds what I'm looking for, your ad stated, 'world cruise to follow.' That's what caught my eye, that and the free room and board."

"Yes, well, I have a seventy-foot wood motor sailor that I recently purchased. Everything under the water line is in excellent shape; there is no dry rot, cracks, or leaks. All the mechanical equipment function perfectly, it's above the waterline; the superstructure, the staterooms, the heads, the galley, the helm, and everything else! The sails, masts, booms; everything, the cleats, mooring lines, portholes, and all the electronics… you name it, it all needs work!"

"A year's worth of labor and tech work, including wiring, plumbing, rigging, painting, oiling, and scraping. Does that fancy your interest?"

"A year's worth of work fancy's my interest. I left my job as a naturalist two years ago and been just bumming around ever since. Waiting tables, working in a dive shop, spending my savings, nothing serious. I jog, swim, lift weights, eat healthy, and smoke a cigarette every now and then."

"I'm almost forty-four years old so the room and board sounds attractive as well. I've been living with my mom and dad for quit some time and that's getting touchy."

"The wage I offer is not much, a hundred bucks a week, its spending money. The room and board would make up for the lack of cash, and it will get you out of the house." "The work is hands and knees as you well know, squatting, bending, sanding, painting, oils, all the bad stuff that goes with a wood boat."

"The forward mast is twenty-eight feet tall, have you ever been up in a boson's-chair?"

"I never have, but I can handle the sails and rigging, if you show me the way I'm sure I can handle the boson's chair."

"The job is just a matter of getting up each day and going to work. Four or five hours a day or you can work as long as you like, but the pay is still the same. I'll be working as well, I need to know the boat inside and out, stern to bow, port to starboard, and working it is the way I learn."

"The person I hire for this job will become the first mate when the cruise starts."

"Can I look at the boat?"

"By all means, can you meet me tonight on D dock, slip 903, around six?"

"Sure."

Johnny and Stella shake hands for the second time.

Through the course of the conversation, Johnny learned Stella had come from a long line of seafarers, seamanship was in her blood. Her grandfather was an officer in the U.S. Navy during both World Wars. Stella's father had a fifty-four-foot Ketch and sailed the globe. Her mother was a rower on the University of Washington NCAA national champion rowing team and was with her father when he sailed the world. Her brother is a Navy Sea-bee.

Stella met Johnny's visual inspection, head-on. She had all the signs of the elements; her skin was brown and weathered from head to toe, and she wore very little cosmetics. Her eyes were clean, clear, alive, and told the story of honest living, high adventure, and hard work. When she shook Johnny's hand, Stella's grip was strong and firm, working muscles, a grip from the body, not just the hand. Stella had spring in her step; she was the real deal.

DH Jimmy had no idea who he was talking to when he approached Sunset Sonny outside The Cobbler Shop, but it was clearly a mistake.

Jimmy was born and raised in Arkansas. His parents, along with his five brothers and sisters, moved to San St. Rosalina when Jimmy was eight years old, except for his four-year hitch in the navy Jimmy has lived there ever since.

Jimmy is now thirty-seven years old, divorced with two kids, and running low on money. He needs to do something, his brothers and sisters, along with numerous nieces, nephews, cousins, and former in-laws live in the city and they keep The Cobbler Shop afloat. The problem is, with most of San St. Rosalina residents and guests in deck oxfords and sandals, the repair business is on the slow burner, and shine business is on the back burner. The Cobbler Shop needs a fix!

"Hi, you're on Fitness for the Day, with Johnny Tucson, how can I help you?"

"Hi Johnny, my name is Lois, and I would like to know what you think of Pilates? My questions for you are; is it good, does it help with balance and coordination, and should I give up going to the weight room and switch to Pilates, what do you think?

"Lois, it depends on what you're looking for. Pilates is more of the teaching of the principals in life, breathing, control, stability, centering yourself. Much different than going into the strength training gym grabbing some steel and pumping it up and down.

In a nutshell, Lois, you will become strong, your range of motion will increase considerably, and your balance and coordination will improve. All this happens while you practice the principles of life, and your muscles will become firm and hard without bulk."

"In the weight room, it's totally different, the majority of the exercisers do progressive resistance, which leads to big and bulk in the muscle department."

"Check this out with a Pilate's instructor, you'll get better and more accurate information then I just gave you. Then go talk with a personal fitness trainer, compare notes, make a decision and go from there."

"Good question, Lois, thank you for calling."

"I really haven't spent much time in a Pilate studio so I cannot answer that question correctly. It is something you have to find out on your own."

"Let me say this, Patsy Cline, remember Patsy Cline, she was a woman in a predominantly man's field. Country music was cowboy music, evolving out on the range with a cow puncher and his harmonica serenading the cows, not many women in that field.

Cowboy music had feeling; there were no electric guitars, horns, pianos, chorus, and mixers, just a feeling coming from the heart and soul. Patsy had that same, 'Come from the heart and soul feeling,' she could sing, and she could feel her way through a song."

"The evolution of Patsy Cline opened the door for Dolly Parton, Tammy Wynette, Taylor Swift, and many of today's great and talented female singers. Much like Billy Jean King did for tennis, and Barbara Walters did for women in television news; pioneers are what they were, someone had to take that first step, and these ladies opened doors."

"In the 1930s through the 1960s, there were very few women in strength training gyms. A person went into a weight room, and it was black steel and men, there were no machines, no cardio equipment, and few women. In the mid-1970s, with the addition of Chapter Nine, all that changed, and the growth of women in sports began."

"High schools and colleges began developing women sports programs. Softball, volleyball, tennis, golf, basketball, and other sports took off like a bat out of the cave, and along with this came strength training.

Machines and cardio equipment join free weights and move into the weight room. Now we have free weights, fixed weights, dumbbells, machines and cardio equipment all under the same roof.

Cory Everson, Rachael McLeish and many other women are opening doors, pink plastic dumbbells, lingerie football, ropes, straps, balls, bands, and tubes. Jane Fonda jumps in with leg warmers and videos, the whole system changes, women supplanted men in sheer numbers."

"Bob Dylan said it, *Them Times they are a Changing*."

"*Heart Like a Wheel*, Shirley Mulroney; remember her of Indy 500 fame?" "I wouldn't be surprised if down the road you'll see a growing number of women in auto racing and a growing number of men in Pilates Studios."

"The Times they *are* a Changing, get out of the way if you can't lend a hand."

"Holy Smokes, land shakes alive, never thought this would happen to me."

"I'm all shook up."

"This is Johnny Tucson coming to you from Radio KETA, 1340, on your FM dial in downtown San St. Rosalina."

"I have Clinton on the line." "Clinton you're on Fitness for a Day with Johnny Tucson; how can I help you?"

"Hi Johnny, I live in Uniontown, Washington, but I'm visiting here in Quiet Cove. I would like to know, in strength training, if you had to choose one lift, what would it be?"

"Clinton, Uniontown, Washington, that's way up there in the Palouse country. I know the neighbor well, born and raised just south of there in Lewiston. Tell me, do they still have that sausage feed?"

"Yes, and it keeps getting bigger every year. More vendors, more eaters, more traffic, and last year they fed over eight thousand people."

"Eight thousand, that's a lot of pigs going to the market!"

"I loved it, breakfast outdoors, black coffee, early morning sunrise, blue skies, miles, and miles of rolling wheat fields, grain silos, and good clean clear fresh air, tough to beat that."

"Of course, things have changed since I was last there, and I've changed as well. Can't remember the last time I ate sausage."

"Clinton, in answer to your question, if I had to choose one lift what would it be, I would choose the old fashion Military Press. Now days I believe they call it the clean and press, but whatever they call it, I just like that exercise. **It requires tension all through the body,**

and Clinton, tension is what builds strength. **Tension** is required in the toes, feet, ankles, and calves, the hams, the gluts, and the quads. **Tension** in the core keeps you rigid; **tension** throughout your back, **tension** in your arms, hands, fingers. Every muscle in your body is called on to play a personal roll."

"It's tough to get any better than that, Clinton, a great all in one lift."

"Others might say the dead lift; others maybe the bench press or the squat. It's a tough call, Clinton, but whatever works for you is right."

"It was good talking to you and bringing back those old memories, Uniontown, Washington, a gas station, a bank, a grocery store, and a school when I was there."

"Thanks for calling."

DH Jimmy usually went down to the Shamrock Room after closing his shop and hashed things over with Carman Fish, but with his finances being the way they are Jimmy hadn't been seen for a few days, today was different. Carman saw Jimmy coming out of the corner of his eye and flipped the cap off a long neck bottle of Bud before Jimmy had a chance to say a word or sit down.

"Long time no see, where you been?" Carman asked, as he slid the Bud in front of Jimmy.

"Been lying low, trying to save a buck or two."

"Has business been that bad you need to cut back on your beer money?"

"It's not booming, if I can hold on until the Gala I believe I could hang in there for another year, see what happens."

"How many shines you do a day?"

"Right now, this time of year I do about four or five, when the Gala starts I'll do about thirty a day. I'll get plenty of other business as well, sandals, heal replacements, a purse or two, handbags; I'm like a lot of small independent merchants, the Christmas season makes or breaks us."

"It's a good thing my ex-wife married wealthy the second time around, if I had to pay child support I never would have never been able to hang in there this long."

"Good for you, Jimmy, my ex's were just the opposite. I made over half-million dollars in four years, and thanks to two marriages, I have nothing to show for it; they took me to the cleaners. That was in Florida, I came west to get a fresh start and hopefully some money ahead, but on a barkeeps wage, I can only hope the tips keep coming my way."

"Maybe we can both marry rich the next time around."

"Ya, maybe, or turn to a life of crime." Carman was setting the stage.

"I definitely need more income," Jimmy said, as he prepared to take a swig of his bottle of Bud.

DH Jimmy always Budweiser Beer and always out of the long neck bottle. He told people "the aroma of the beer filters up my nose while, the taste dribbles down to my throat."

"Ya, don't we all. What are you going to do about it?"

"I don't know, running a business doesn't leave much time for a second job.

Business has been slow, and I mean slow for weeks, not just hours or days. I have to be here, can't just up close and leave for the day, no sir; the sign says open ten to six."

"What kind of money do you need, if its food, gas, or rent money I could help you out?"

"No, I need a steady income twice as much as I'm bringing in now. People aren't repairing shoes like they did in the past; Wal-Mart, Target, Costco make all the money. Folks buy them cheap shoes from the big box then throw 'em away when the soles get thin. In older times people would buy good solid leather shoes, and when the soles wore thin they would resole them, but not these days. And the tennis shoes; wear'm, wash'm, and chuck'm, that's what happens there. The small business owner really has to forge just to stay in business, and then they need a second job to support their personal life."

Stella walked up the gang way of the tramper like it was her God-given right; she was fluid with both hands and both feet. She could turn corners duck her head and bend at the waist without breaking stride. She toured the boat like she had been on board for years, moving through the companionway, up the stairs and around the deck, climbing the mast and hoisting the sails, Stella moved with ease in all manners of motion.

In the wheelhouse, she could read charts, knew the instruments panel, knew celestial navigation, and how to use the sextant. Stella was fluent in Spanish, French, and English; Johnny needed Stella more then she needed him.

Johnny and Stella sit at the makeshift dining table near the stern of the boat.

"Well this is it, what do you think?"

"She's a grand old gal, what make is she?"

"Swedish, Hans Christian, 1960's. Teak, Oak, and Mahogany, all shiplap, countersunk stainless-steel screws, caulk, plugged, and oiled, custom made. Cost a bundle when she was new, I got her for a song and a dance."

Just look at her, Johnny said, rather despondently, "probably could have gotten her for just a song."

"I need a crew of six good sailors to sail around the world with; I'm taking a year off from work for sure, maybe two years, I need a change in my life, I've been working at the radio station too long. I need to have some excitement and adventure in my life, go to new countries, spend a month or two in different ports then move on. I'm looking for other people who have that same feeling."

"I'm going to need a shipwright, an engineer/mechanic, a navigator and I'll need a cook, but today, well, you see it, scraping, painting, cleaning, are you interested?"

"Yes, of course, boaters are always working their boat. The boat is outside in the water, wind, rain, and sun all day every day; it always needs to be worked on, cleaning, scrubbing, scraping, painting. Equipment must always be inspected and in excellent working condition. Everything must be battened down, lines checked, no frayed, knots secured, cleats fasten tight."

"No matter who you are, on the water everyone helps in maintaining the boat. You can't just pull over and call triple-A. It's a way of life on the high seas, if you can't do maintenance you don't belong on the water."

"Isn't that the truth?"

"Well, this is what it's about. I need the elbow work today; skullduggery is down the road."

Stella was nodding her head, smiling, agreeing, chipping in a, "yes," "I understand," "sure," "completely," whenever the opportunity presented itself. Johnny rambled on.

"All of us will need to work to raise expense money as we travel; we'll pay as we go. We'll do whatever it takes to earn this money, unload freight, box bananas, cut cane, mend sails, repair nets, whatever, as long as it is legal."

"I'm about a year away from sailing; you can live onboard, work twenty to twenty-five hours a week. I'll supply all the equipment, including food, and give you one hundred dollars cash every Friday. In other words, it's free room and board plus the money for twenty to twenty-five hours of work a week. And, because you will know the boat through and through, you will become the first mate when the cruse begins.

"It isn't much cash for a person with your skill level, but then again, you could get a second part-time job and still have your room and board and part-time job here plus be a part of the trip."

"The job is yours if you want it. Let me give you a day or two to think it over."

"No, that's not necessary, Johnny, I've already made up my mind, I'll take the job."

"Thank you so much," Stella said, as she extended her hand in the same breath, thus not giving Johnny a chance to back out.

"As you said," "it gets me out of the house."

Excitement filled the air!

"I have been around the world twice; I know ports where we can get work. I know people who can get us work; I know good secure routes, safe havens, no pirates."

"I know tides, currents, when's the best time to set sail and when to lay up."

Now it was Stella's turn to ramble on.

"There are plenty of young kids out there who have fat bank accounts, compliments of their parents. They pay good money for passage from one continent to another; I know how to locate these kids. I know boats, I'm a journeyman sailor."

"When do I start," Stella asked, as she was laughing, smiling, feeling the excitement of a new and long-awaited adventure, entering into her life.

"Ha, welcome aboard," Johnny said, smiling.

Johnny and Stella were shaking hands for the third time that day.

"Stow your gear in one of the staterooms; find another to call home, and start there. I have all the equipment in the hole." "How about some dinner to celebrate, I'm buying."

"Sounds great to me, I'm starving."

"You can use the captain's quarters to freshen up."

As soon as Stella was out of sight, Johnny began jumping up and down, pumping his fist, smiling and thinking how lucky he is to have a shipmate like Stella.

"Hi, you're on Fitness for the Day, with Johnny Tucson; what can I help you with Anne?"

"Hi Johnny, I love your program. I listen to you as often as I can. The question I have for you is: sometimes I'm running short on time are there one or two exercises I can do when I'm in a hurry?"

"Anne, there are several exercises to do when you're short on time. Do the squat, the dead lift, or the clean and press. Do any one of these, ten reps, two sets, and you're good to go. These lifts will activate the major muscles in your body, and work multiple joints as well."

"You can also do circuit training, Anne."

"Most gyms have a stationary circuit set up where you go from one station to another with no rest in between. These stations are set up in such a way that when you complete the circuit your entire muscular system is worked, as well as the cardiopulmonary system.

It takes about twenty-thirty minutes to complete the circuit, than you're out the door."

"Good question, Anne, thanks for calling."

DH Jimmy had been a star football player at Union High School in San St. Rosalina. At five feet ten inches tall and one hundred eighty pounds, Jimmy was muscle head to toe. Offensive linemen do not often receive avocation for being a star but not so in his case. Jimmy played three years of varsity and was credited with twenty-seven pancake blocks. He was a terror on the field, threw his body around with reckless disregard. Three times he was flagged for unnecessary roughness after tackling the defensive backs on interceptions.

Jimmy played with broken fingers, a broken nose; he was the first player on the practice field and the last one off. College scholarships poured in, but college was not in his plans, Jimmy was blue collar at heart, a man skilled to work with his with hands, back, and feet.

After his four-year hitch in the navy, Jimmy returned home, married his high school sweetheart, and eight months into the marriage, a baby boy was on the way. It was time for Jimmy to find some serious work. He was a sonar tech in the navy, but working inside a steel hull with headsets was not his cup of tea.

One day while visiting a friend's workshop, Jimmy found his calling. Standing around, shooting the breeze, Jimmy picked up the small cobbler's hammer and liked the feel. The nails were small, but even with his deformed fingers Jimmy could place them where he wanted. The work was nice; it was light, no heavy lifting or loud noise and the leather felt smooth, soft, and comfortable in his hands.

His friends said it paid a living, but like any business, it needed to be worked. Jimmy inquired about serving an apprenticeship with no wage, the deal was set. For thirteen weeks, Jimmy worked side by side with Steve Lo, five hours a day, five days a week, finally, the mall opened, Jimmy put money down on The Cobbler Shop.

Cameron Blue was not going anywhere with his life, and that's the way he wanted it; running the elevator at the Ruby Rose Hotel is where he wanted to be. He showed up every morning at five-thirty for his six o'clock shift. He didn't wear a uniform, but he always looked spiffy; clean-shaven, hair nicely combed, fingernails clipped and clean, shoes shined, and clothing neatly pressed. Cameron is intelligent, personable, and friendly; all this added up to a good fit for the job.

Although Cameron was only thirty-six years old, the prognosis for him was a kidney transplant. A genetic thing handed down from generation to generation. His grandfather passed at thirty-six, his father at forty, and his brother at forty-three all from kidney failure. The hotel had insurance for Cameron, but not for this; major medical was not included. Then there was the waitlist, these issues had been on the back of Cameron's mind for the past few years; now they were at the forefront.

"Hello, you're on Fitness for the Day with Johnny; how can I help you?"

"Hi Johnny, my name is Ruth; I am calling from San St. Rosalina. What is the best to use, free weights or machines?"

"Good morning, a pleasure to take your call today. I would say use them both, Ruth, in fact, get to know every piece of equipment in the gym." "Sooner or later you will narrow things down to what you like to use best."

"Some of the equipment you will use more than others but get to know how every piece of equipment in the gym works. Free weights, fixed weights, dumbbells, machines, circuit training, Bosh balls, tubes, bands, mirrors; every piece of equipment is there for purpose and they all have something to offer."

"I will say this, Ruth; with free weights you can create your own line of travel, whereas with machines they travel on a fixed line. Also, with the free weights you can stand and use the mirrors, which help with balance, core and posture."

"Thanks for calling."

"Let me remind everyone, Tony (Rock'n) Rowland, will be with us on the twentieth of the month, so be sure to call in. Tony has been appearing at the station for the past four years, and he is very open as to what he talks about, family life, music, and life on the road, you name it. Tony (Rock'n) Rowland, ten forty-five on the twentieth."

Big Bill is Etta's long-time partner. Bill is bigger than Etta by a bunch, but Etta is still the boss. Bill is in charge of all the security and property maintenance surrounding the restaurant from the beginning of the park through the offices. His security force employs thirty-seven people and operates twenty-four hours a day. Nobody carries a sidearm, but they each carry a small can of pepper spray in their pocket. They wear headsets, which keep them in constant contact with one another. The security force also includes twenty-six cameras, which are monitored twenty-four-seven.

Bill also oversees the eight-member park staff. From the parking lot to the front door of Etta's is four hundred and sixty-eight feet as the crow flies. The ten-foot-wide flagstone walkway does not fly like the crow; it meanders slightly and has forks leading through the gardens. The park includes the Polish hot dog vending cart and its landscape, three gazebos, a twenty-four foot, and a twelve-foot arbor, four fountains, two ponds, the herb gardens, the flower and veggie gardens; light fixtures, tables, benches, the restaurant, and the restrooms.

Nine electric golf carts, which are shared among maintenance, security, and valet parking, are also under Bill's supervision, as are the business offices behind the restaurant. Upstairs above the business offices is where Radio KETA is located; this is where Johnny Tucson broadcasts, "Fitness for the Day."

"Hi, you're on Fitness for the Day with Johnny; how can I help you?"

"Hi Johnny, my name is Clark, I'm calling from Quiet Cove. Can you explain what, 'drop sets', are?"

"Good morning, Clark, sure, I can tell you about drop sets. You make the resistance lighter while you increase the reps. For example; let's say you are going to do the dumbbell curl, standing in front of the dumbbell rack, you pick up two forty-pound dumbbells, do six reps, set the forty's down and pick up two thirty-five pounders, do eight reps, set the thirty-five pounders down and pick up two thirty-pounders do ten reps, and so on until you work to failure. Again, you lower the resistance while you increase the reps; there is no rest between sets."

Tension begins with your first rep, Clark, not you're second, third, or fourth. Your muscles are on fire when you finish, you'll 'feel the burn.'

"Did I make myself clear on that, Clark?"

"Yes you did, Johnny, I'm going to try drop sets when I go to the gym tomorrow. What if I'm on the bench press?"

"Start heavy and have a partner remove the weights as you go through the sets, just remember, 'increase the reps, lower the resistance, no rest.' A great way to strength train, thanks for calling, Clark."

"Good morning and welcome to Fitness for the Day; I'm Johnny Tucson how can I help?"

"Hi Johnny, thanks for taking my call, I'm Michael from San St. Rosalina. Will you please tell me a good way to keep your lower back loose?"

"Michael, I like the old fashion way, stand with your feet together, knees straight but not locked, bend down from the waist and touch your toes. This stretch doesn't stretch the back muscle, but it will open up the hamstrings, gluts, and calves, which allows for greater flexibility on your backside."

"A great stretch, been around for years, try it, see what you think. I do it six or ten times a day, it's very simple and easy." "Do it at the bank while you're standing in line."

"Good question, Michael, and remember, engage your core and go slow into and slow out of the stretch, with your head coming up last."

Hi, this is radio 1340 on your FM dial, Fitness for the Day with Johnny Tucson; how may I help you?

"Hi Johnny, my name is Rachael; I'm calling from San St. Rosalina. Will you please tell me when to inhale, and exhale, when lifting weights?"

"Sure, of course, Rachael. There are always two parts to any strength exercise, exertion, and relaxation. A person inhales during the relaxation phase of the exercise, fills up the lungs with good fresh oxygenated air, and then exhales during the exertion phase of the exercise.

"For example, Rachael, if you were doing the bench press, inhale while you are lowering the bar to your chest, filling up the lungs with fresh oxygen than exhale while you're pushing the bar up. 'Inhale during relaxation, exhale during exertion,' are we good on this, Rachael?"

"Yes, I believe so, inhale when you relax and exhale when you exert, that's simple enough to remember."

"Very good, Rachael, what a great question, most beginners get confused over this, when to inhale and when to exhale when doing weight lifting. Believe me when I say, proper breathing techniques are important. Thanks for the call, Rachael."

At twenty-nine years old, Charmain Green had been divorced twice; her Master's Degree in English has been sitting on the shelf for five years. Charmain has plenty of bounce in her step and is looking to crank her life up a notch or two. Today is Charmain's day off, she and Carman Fish are having dinner together.

"I don't know," Charmain answered, "I always seem to pick the wrong guy. I keep thinking of Troy Barting, he wanted to marry me out of high school, but I said no. Troy is the tall, dark, handsome type, good grades in school, president of the senior class, college-bound, and all the good stuff. Today he is a successful banker living with his wife and two small children in Scottsdale, Arizona, a success story for sure. I could have been Mrs. Troy Barting, instead, I pick Ronnie Rudmyre and Tom Fisher, and here I am waiting tables and singing the, "Car Wash Blues."

"But you know, I wasn't ready for marriage out of high school, actually I'm not ready for marriage today. It's obvious, two ex-husbands and I'm not even thirty years old."

"I know where you're coming from, been there done that. Some people are just not made for marriage; I'm in no hurry to find wife number three I'll tell you that."

"Have you always been a bartender?"

"No, I've been into big money, and that's where I would like to get back too. It takes a lot of money to live in America today, thirty, forty, thousand dollars a year doesn't cut it anymore. If a person wants to raise a family, it takes a zillion dollars. If a person likes to travel, go places, see the world, learn a different culture, speak a different language, it takes somewhat less, but that's the type of person

I am. I don't want to be the fish in the tank all my life just for three squares a day and the safety and security of home, you know what I mean."

Charmain acknowledges that she knew what Carman meant.

"I'm looking for ways to come up with some really big money. Working for a wage doesn't cut it these days unless you have several college degrees and degrees on top of those degrees."

Carman Fish was a drug smuggler, not a gun runner. He never packed a gun; he never used a gun, in fact, Carman never owned a gun. He didn't want to spend a lifetime in prison if a dishonest job went south, and not having a gun was the best way to achieve this.

Carman was planning to burglarize the Ruby Rose Hotel on New Year's Eve night, the night of the Gala Invitational. A gun was not in the plan, and the plan was simple, an inside job.

Carman's life of crime began at an early age; he would steal pens from fellow students while in grade school and give them to his buddies from other schools in hopes of cashing in on future I O U's. In middle school, he began taking books out of the library and selling them to friends. In high school, it was the same, books, athletic equipment, and term papers. It wasn't big money, but it was easy money, and it beat mowing lawns and raking leaves.

Carman didn't need to steal, his father was a lawyer, and his mother was a teacher. Genetically speaking, Carman was handsome, smart, and well-groomed, but he had been smitten by a life of crime at an early age, and it carried with him during his later years.

At age fourteen, Carman stole a car and drove from Miami Beach to Winter Haven before he ran into a tree. The officer on the scene was about to take Carman to the station house when suddenly Carman bolted. Young and fast-a-foot, Carman knew he could outrun the officer, who now at the age of fifty-something was overweight, slow, and in no condition to give chase beyond a few hundred yards. Carman was making up a story while talking to his father over the phone as to why he needed a ride home from Winter Haven.

This little escapade would have gone unnoticed except for the fact three weeks later the officer in charge was vacationing in Miami Beach. Carman had his mug plastered on the seventh page of the Miami Herald for throwing a well-pitched baseball and knocking out the red/blue emergency flasher lights of a Dade County Sheriff's car.

The vacationing officer recognized Carman immediately, who else had a blue Mohawk haircut with a long earring dangling from his ear. Carman was never charged with grand thief auto but was cited for, The Pitch, as it became known in the Miami area.

Carman's life of crime continued on the upswing. At age seventeen, he and his girlfriend walked into a jewelry store in Fort Lauderdale looking for an engagement ring. While the clerk was busy with Carman two of Carman's friends enter the store, the clerk called for assistance. Minutes later, two single women, also friends of Carman enter the store at separate times, six people, two clerks; it was easy for Carman to switch the fake ring for the real one.

Carman sold the ring to a fence; he and his buddies split a grand. Not bad for a few hours of fun and work.

At age nineteen, Carman enrolled at the University of Miami to study criminology. While there, he took rock climbing, strength training, and balance classes. It was the eleventh floor, always the eleventh floor; the Cat Burglar was leaving a signature. Well over three years have passed since the last snatch, and no one had seen or heard of the Cat Burglar since, but suspicion traveled about. Carman Fish wore number eleven on this football jersey; he also wore number eleven on his baseball uniform.

Roxanne Rodriquez was not considered high maintenance, but she could be. Long raven black hair, huge brown eyes, and at five feet four she had curves in all the right places, the men just loved Roxy. The guys Roxy hung with already had two children of their own, along with a wife, a house, and a mortgage. Roxy knew this, but they were fun and not interested in marriage.

Aside from having excellent physical characteristics, Roxy had brains; she earned her way. She finished secretarial school eight years back and was working as such at the Ruby Rose Hotel when Viola Washington, the hotel CEO, offered Roxy the position of personal secretary. Roxy obliged, and for the past two years Roxanne Rodriquez has been sitting at the right hand of Viola Washington.

"Good morning and welcome to Fitness for the Day; I'm Johnny Tucson, how can I help you?"

"Hi Johnny, my name is Mike, I live in Harbor Town. I like your program, it is very informative, and I like the music you spin. I'm calling today to ask about the bicep curl, one friend tells me I should move my entire arm when I do the curl while another says I should just move the forearm. Which friend is correct?"

"Mike, if it is just the bicep muscle you're looking to work just bend the elbow; do not use the upper arm. Tuck your elbows into your rib cage; with the elbows planted hard against the ribs it's easy to isolate the upper arm. If you're not tucked in, a person tends to use the upper arm. Mike, you can also use the bicep curl machine. Thanks for calling."

"I would like to remind everyone about Etta's, tonight, hot Disc Jock Carl Alexander will be spinning the records. If you like to dance you'll love this, from seven o'clock to midnight. Carl spins everything from oldies but goodies to a big swing band, rock' roll, rap, hip hop, and even throws in a little country. There's something for everyone no matter your age or genre, Carl Alexander."

"Put on your dancing shoes and hit the hardwood tonight at Etta's for a good night of fun, food, and music."

Roxy was a divorced soccer mom and had one boy age six, and one girl age eight. She was an outstanding mother, aside from work she was usually there for her children. She was home at six, dinner at seven, homework, TV, and bed by nine. Roxanne had to have fun too, and her children knew this and were very happy when grandma and granddad came to baby sit. However, something was missing from Roxy's life and she couldn't put her finger on it. The children were there, money was there, friends were there, the support system was in place, and men were handy, but there was a void inside Roxy's heart.

Carman Fish and Roxy were work buddies. They would have lunch together; sometimes they had lunch with Charmain, maybe with Cameron and Jimmy, sometimes all four. Carman Fish is cultivating his friendship; he is, in fact, *the straw that stirs the drink.*

Roxy found it a pleasure sharing a meal with Carman. When he told stories from his Miami days about the 'Cat Burglar', the person who crawled, in the darkness of night time eleven stories up the side of a high-rise condo, hand over hand, foot over foot, with nothing to hold onto except window ledges, rain gutters, and deck rails, Roxy's adrenaline would just spike.

Other times there were the drug-running stories. Racing across the Gulf of Mexico during the midnight hour at speeds up to ninety miles an hour outrunning the law, these stories left Roxy breathless. Carman always made the stories exciting and beyond the call of life, and of course he never mentioned he was the leading character in the episodes.

It was the thrill of putting it all on the line Roxy though, your life for gold, success or death, no in between, what a thrill.

Excitement! That was the missing element in the soccer mom's heart.

The arcade games at Etta's have been lit up all day. The pool tables were stacked with money, the DJ was spinning records, dancers were dancing, diners were dining, alcohol was flowing, and all is well.

Etta and Big Bill had a suite at the Ruby Rose Hotel reserved year-round, their clothes hung there, the bathroom was full, and the refrigerator had cheese and wine . Running Etta's was a full-time job and more; sometimes Etta and Bill didn't feel like driving home after a long day on the job, the Ruby Rose was home away from home.

Their suite was a corner unit on the third floor overlooking Sunset Bay Marina; it was quiet, peaceful, and comfortable. Often times in the quiet and darkness of the wee hours in the morning, Etta and Bill would take a stroll down to the marina. It was an old marina, wood creosote piles with wood catwalks anchored to them. The lighting was dim and the shadows were tall, dark, and sparse, quiet and stillness filled the early morning air.

The workboats and pleasure crafts tied to the mooring cleats had their own look, size, and personalities. Etta and Bill would smile at the boats and talk to them as if they were alive, they would talk about them, and point out striking, funny, amazing, and fancy features these boats possessed. They would try to guess the name of the boat and how much that boat would cost, and they would guess where that boat could take them in this old world. This was fun for Etta and Bill, they never tired of it.

The smell of the salt sea air was refreshing to them. It was a nostalgic place for Etta taking her back to the days of her father and grandfather. The docks had been here forty years, and Etta saw the first piles being hammered into the mud and watched as the marina grew into what is today. Yesteryear's stores had sprung up along the shoreline with plank board walkways. The stores, like the boats, had their own personality, some with old cedar siding, others with shake shingles, while others were made of stucco.

There were fishing stores, marine hardware stores, an eatery, a harbor master's building with toilets and showers for seafarers, realtor's offices, boat sales offices, dive shops, clothing stores, and much more. Window shopping is what they called it. Etta and Bill would walk along the boardwalk and look at the displays in the windows, see if there were any changes from the last time they passed and what new fashions were on display. At this hour in the morning, they would be the only people on the boardwalk.

The walk was rejuvenating for them and took their mind off business as well as the hustle and bustle of the daily activities life. This was their time, quiet time, and they used it well.

Neither Etta nor Bill are billionaires, but they wouldn't have trouble writing a check for a hundred grand or two. Because Etta is who she is, her and Bill had an open invite to the Gala Invitational, they have attended every one.

Freighters arriving from various ports throughout the world lay anchor in Sunset Bay until it was time to move up the waterway to the unloading docks. A launch from Sunset Bay Marina shuttles the crew back and forth from the anchored ships to the marina. When they arrived at the marina the first place the sailors stopped was Etta's.

Etta, as pretty and wealthy as she is, is no stranger to the blue-collar world. Having worked hand and hand with her father on the fishing boat, Etta could get down in the mud with the sailors and hold her own. When the crew walked into the restaurant, Etta was the first person with a big smile, an extended hand, and a hardy welcome.

She knew the crew had been away from home for quite some time, and there was nothing like a home away from home. Eggs and bacon any time, the steaks were thick and juicy, potatoes were Idaho Russets, which meant big and baked. Spaghetti and meatballs were the house specialty, and the whiskey was strong. The sailors loved Etta's!

When the sailors ordered a pie, they didn't order a slice of pie, they ordered the whole pie. Coffee came in the pot, not a cup. Often time Etta and Big Bill would be hob-knobbing with the crew, going from table to table sharing pie and coffee, laughing, joking, and enjoying the moment. Even though the sailors didn't understand English and Etta and Bill didn't speak their language, they did what they did, and it couldn't get any better.

When Etta hosted the Seaman's Christmas Special, she coughed up the two to three thousand dollars that feed every soul with a seaman's card. Even if a person wasn't packing a seaman card there was plenty of turkey, mash potatoes, dressing, and the like to go around. Etta did things for the good of the community, and it was also good for business; excellent customer relations, good food, and friendly service are what made Etta's the West Coasts' answer to the Statute of Liberty.

"Did you stop at Etta's?" world travelers would ask."

Stella had her room looking new in no time. Johnny told her at the outset that twenty to twenty-five hours a week was all she was asked to work, but she put her nose to the grindstone and did the job sooner than expected. The room was scraped, sanded, and oiled; a new shower curtain was hung, light fixtures were clean and polished, the portholes were cleaned and polished, inside as well as outside. The floor was looking clean and bright, and a new mattress was on the bed.

"Do you like it," Stella asked?

"Yes, excellent, outstanding job, and you've added some color,"

"Some white with a little yellow trim, I thought I would add some color to break up the all-wood look. We can use the same colors for each room, just break up the pattern."

"Very impressive," Johnny answered, as he stepped inside to take a closer look. The head was complete, the mirror was shining, towel fixtures were polished, the closet was finished, new webbing was hung, it couldn't have been any better, Johnny thought.

"Did you tape off the transitions?"

"No, I freehanded all the way, I used Basso on the windows, and I even used it on the chrome, it did a wonderful job."

"It sure did, and so did you, what a highlight, how outstanding!"

"Everything is dry; I thought I would move my gear in today and start on the next room tomorrow."

"Sounds good to me, how about a Polish, I'm buying?"

"I'm accepting!"

Stella and Johnny take a table next to the vendor's stand. The day is warm and the sky is blue and sunny. Johnny has mustard, sauerkraut, and relish on his Polish, Stella is eating hers with mustard. A gentleman sits at the table next to them and starts talking about the Polish sausage.

"I like to eat Polish sausage twice a month. I'm into good health, over the years I've given up sugar foods, greasy foods, pizzas, and breads but will never give up my Polish, along with its condiments of course."

"In Poland, you can order the sausage fried, smothered in fried onions, stewed, or supped. Here in America, we Americans always eat it like it's a hot dog, put it in a bun, load it with your favorites, and chomp away. Anyway you eat it, it's good."

"I like it," Johnny replied, "I come here quite often; I always eat it with mustard, relish, and sauerkraut. The Polish sausage is good enough that someday it may crowd the hot dog out of, 'Baseball, Hot Dogs, and Apple Pie.'"

"You think someday it might be, 'Baseball, Polish Sausage, and Apple Pie?'"

"Well, maybe not, but the Polish is good."

"Funny thing, the Polish sausage is actually from Poland, but French toast isn't from France, it's from Belgium."

"And the French fry, where is that from?" Stella added.

"The fry has been around for a long time, the stranger answered, no one really knows where the fry calls home."

The stranger is tall, handsome, and well-mannered, has good posture, and wore fine cloth. He spoke with a southern accent like maybe Mississippi or Tennessee.

"Where are you from?"

I'm from Florida, the stranger replied, "Maybe about three thousand miles from here. The sunshine is the same, the sky is the same, the sand is different, but the Polish sausage, with mustard sauerkraut and relish, tastes the same, just as good there as it is here."

"Are you here on business?"

"No, I moved here about a year and a half ago; I work right there," the stranger said, as he pointed to the Ruby Rose Hotel, "I'm the bartender in the Shamrock Room."

On December twenty-ninth, the Ruby Rose Hotel will host billionaires from all around the world for four days of fun, excitement, and **down-home living**. On the twenty-ninth and for the next three days, all one hundred and fourteen rooms in the hotel will be reserved for the Sixth Annual Billionaires Gala Invitational Ball. Private charter boats have reserved slips in Sunset Bay Marina as close to the hotel as they can get.

Fishing boats, pleasure crafts, touring boats, and seaplanes line the harbor's edge. Everyone is in line; the services are free to the billionaires, paid for out of their five-thousand-dollar invitation fee, it's the big tip money the boaters are after; friendly service, good days of fishing, smiles, handshakes, high fives, good beer, and excellent whiskey can fetch a grand or two a day in tip money.

The attire for the four-day Gala is sandals or the like, shorts and open shirts for the men, and casual wear for the women. Anyone caught wearing formal attire during the day-light hours will spend a sixty-minute lunch break in the hoosegow.

The hoosegow is a make-shift jail set up by the hotel where offenders of the dress code are fingerprinted, mugged, and placed on public display behind iron bars. Other partygoers walk by and offer up peanuts or a hamburger off the value menu.

Photographs of the jailbirds are on display throughout the Gala. There are several offenders every year, but never any two-time offenders. When the Gala committee says casual, they want casual, this is **down-home living time.** In the evening, the partiers can wear what they choose.

Etta's gets plenty of runoff from the Gala. When these wealthy folks stroll into Etta's, their pockets are filled with fives, tens, and twenty-dollar bills, which they quickly converted into quarters at the change machines. The quarters are for the arcade games. The pinball machines stay lit up for three days and nights, the only break here is when management stops the game to empty the quarters. The lines are long at the shuffleboard tables as well; singles, doubles, or mixed, take your pick at ten quarters a game it's a bargain.

The Indy Five Hundred is a biggie as well; here two drivers sit side by side in makeshift Indy cars. An overhead television screen monitors their driving as they go boom, crash, bang, and ting-a-ling into the walls and other cars as they try to out jostle each other to the finish line. Just finishing the race is a laugh and a high five.

Pool is an international game; The Greeks can be seen playing with the Brazilians, the Columbians with the Russians, the British with the Scots, and the Americans with anyone. The wager is the same for eight ball, rotation, singles, doubles or mixed, two twenty's on the table, the winner takes all.

Everyone, regardless of sex, race, age, or nationality, can be seen with cue in hand, eating, drinking, laughing, and talking about the days when they were the hotshot pool shark down at the local watering hole. Darts, ping pong, horseshoes, it's all there.

The clock ticks on, quarters keep on dropping, night turns into day, day turns into night, the laughter and fun keep on keep'n on.

When the men hit the fishing boats and arcade games, the women hit the shopping mall. Spas, mud baths, nail salon, buying sandals, handbags, sunglasses, spending is what they came to do, and spending is what they're going to do.

A gal walks into, "**Rita's, the New You,**" two hours later she emerges from the same door, gray hair is now red with green and black streak**s**. Red lipstick has given way to hot pink, and two earrings replace one.

Plain-Jane toe nails are red, white, and blue with rhinestone sandals onboard each foot, toe rings ascent it all. Head up, chest out, shoulders back, "I like the new you," she proudly proclaims.

Not into a new doo, "**Tuck A Way,**" is the place to shop. Hats of all sizes, shapes, and colors are found there. Beanies, baseball caps, cowgirl hats, straw hats, berets, add a new stash, accent it with fancy sunglasses, and Jane is now, Lamoure.

But it's the "High Ball" the gals love best. Around the corner and down the street from the Ruby Rose Hotel sits the High Ball, a single-story seventy thousand square foot gaming building where Champaign and wine are on the house, hard not to like that.

Crap tables, roulette wheels, Black Jack tables, Texas Hold'm, five-card draw, stud, and spin the wheel tables are everywhere. Slot machines, with real American nickels dimes and quarters bring screams, shouts, and laughter when the bells and whistles blast off and those real American coins tingle down into those new beanies and caps.

Salad bars, sandwich shops, cheesecake booths, bagel bars, fried pies, and chocolate sundae eating salons circle the perimeter. Eat what you want, drink while you're here, and play all night long.

The Champaign, and wine keep on flowing, and the party keeps on going. Can it get any better? I don't think so. Uncork another bottle of Champaign; ninety-eight bottles of Champaign on the shelf, take one down pass it around, ninety-seven bottles of Champaign.....

Any time and any place in the city the billionaires can be seen dancing in the streets. Taxi cabs are pulled off to the side of the road, windows rolled down, doors wide open, and music blasting out into the midwinter air. The big swingers and the hot babes are doing the swing and loving every minute of it.

Guys and gals can be seen sitting on bar stools eating and drinking, expressing to each other how the simple times in life passed them by.

Some of these folks had family money to help get them started. After Harvard, Yale, Cambridge, or Oxford, there was law school or a masters in finance then onto the family business. For others, it was the clock after graduate school, they went to work in the office, where the nine to five became nine until midnight.

Whatever the case, there were no street hoops, no city parks department pick-up games, no local YMCA's or Boys/Girls Club for these folks there were no Levis, sweatshirts, and tennis shoes. For them it was, 'The Club', wing-tip shoes, button-down shirts, three-piece suits, and sailboats. It was high heel shoes, nylon stockings, fancy dresses, debutants, and *high income* marriages.

The Gala Invitational takes these folks back in time, picking up those years they missed in the parks. Their legs are stiff and their arms don't stretch like they use to; but they can still dribble, shoot, hit, run, throw, yell, scream, scrape their elbows, knees, and bleed red blood. Their hearts and desires fuel them beyond their imagination, beads of sweat pour from their face and drench their shirts, but you know what, they love it!

"Make-up, we don't need no stinking make-up."

"I tell you it's foolproof," Carman Fish is telling the others, as he unveiled his plan to rob the Ruby Rose Hotel. Gathered around Carman are DH Jimmy, Cameron Blue, and Charmain Green. "The chances of getting caught are about as great as winning the lottery."

Carman eggs on, "Cameron just said nobody ever leaves the party until well after midnight, and he's been on the job five years. This leaves us a good hour and thirty minutes to get the job done." Carman Fish was a good judge of character, he cultivated his friendship with this group of people out of two dozen or so folks he developed friendships with. Jimmy and Cameron both need money, Carman wasn't sure what was on Charmain's mind, but he felt he could confide in her.

It took Carman months of breakfast, lunch, and dinner money, brain-teasing, what if's, make-believes, and imaginary spending to get this far. He revealed his plan to these three people because he felt sure he could trust them, they saw the light. Every time a room was vacated in the hotel, the key card was changed, as was the combination to the safe.

On December twenty-eighth, all rooms in the hotel would be vacated, cleaned, aired and dressed. The billionaires would be arriving on the twenty-ninth, this meant Roxanne Rodriquez had one day to hack into the CEO's computer and steal the combinations to the safes. Once the combinations and key cards were in hand, the rest was simple.

Carman and Charmain would take their lunch break at ten-thirty on New Year's Eve night. They would hook up with DH Jimmy and Gulf Coast Bill at the main elevator, conveniently operated by Cameron Blue. For security reasons, this was the only elevator operating on New Year's Eve night. All stairwell doors were locked as well as all security exits; they could only be opened remotely by a switch at the front desk, by Cameron Blue, or by management. There would be no one allowed on floors two and three without an escort.

"Earlier," Carman went on, Cameron said that in the past no one had left the party until well after midnight maybe around one or two in the morning, but that doesn't mean it will not happen in the future. Each of us will wear a headset, which will enable you to hear and speak to the others. If someone leaves the party to go back to their room for some reason, Cameron will ask that person which room they would like. We'll hear the answer and take appropriate action."

Under no circumstances were the thieves to take anything that was not in the safe, even if it was a diamond necklace. This ruling was capitalized, headlined, and underscored by Carman. "If someone should come back looking for something and it wasn't in sight, they would go to the safe, which may have already been looted."

"Hi, you're on Fitness for the Day with Johnny; how can I help you?

"Hi Johnny, my name is Meg, I'm from San St. Rosalina. I would like to know how often a person should change their routine."

"Good question, Meg; a person should change their routine every six to eight weeks. Routines become stale, boring, and your muscles will adapt, change everything, not just the reps and sets. For example, if you've been doing the bench press for some time switch to the dumbbell fly, it works the same muscles only with a wider range of motions and from a different angle."

"If you're doing the triceps kickback, do the triceps pull down. Mix it up, Meg, there are a lot of muscles in the human body and most can all be worked from different angles while achieving the same goals. Every six to eight weeks, Meg, thanks for calling."

DH Jimmy had a lot on his mind. When Jimmy was in the navy, his shoes had the best shine of all the sailors on board ship. He was proud of his shine and was always receiving compliments about them; he stood tall on inspection day. Jimmy carried his gifted talent over into civilian life, and with much of the same fanfare, people loved his spit shine. His marketing plan was simple. He charged sixteen dollars per spit shine figuring the customer would give him a twenty dollar bill and tell him to keep the change, and that is what usually happened. Jimmy would bring in about $100 a day on shines, multiply that by six days a week, and this money was supposed to be 'extra' money. As it turned out, this money was money Jimmy counted on to pay the bills, there was no 'extra' money.

Most of the shoppers in the mall were women and Jimmy was trying to figure out how he could tap into that market. He would mend a handbag every now and again, he fixed broken high heel shoes, shined mid-knee boots, but the pickings were slim and he was in a high rent district. On this day, pedicures entered his mind. Why not, Jimmy thought, if he could tap into that source he could easily double or triple his income. Jimmy reached for the phone; he called his friend Rosalie to discuss pedicures.

Rosalie, who owns a salon on San St. Rosalina's east side, was quite surprised when Jimmy told her what he was thinking.

"DH Jimmy, my God, I'm doing fine, how are you? Marie's birthday, it's been that long since we've talked, two months, good to hear your voice."

"I'm doing fine, Rosalie, yes it has been a while. I've been meaning to call you, but this happened, that happened, time slips by, and before you know it, it's like you said, two months."

"Rosalie, I'm looking to expand my business, its advice, and a lunch date I'm calling you about."

"The lunch date I can do, what kind of advice are you looking for?"

"I'm thinking of going into the pedicure business, a small add on to The Cobbler Shop. Most of the shoppers in the mall are women, and I thought maybe I would go in that direction. There is a pedicure shop here in the mall and every time I walk by its full. What's your take on this?"

"Pedicures! The booming right guard on the high school football team, well, whatever pays the bills, right Jimmy?"

"Yap, right, "you got to do what you got to do."

"I will say this, Jimmy, the pedicure business is booming, we gals like to pamper ourselves, and the feet take the burden of the beat down. We wear sandals quite often and we want our feet to not only feel good but to look nice. What do you have in mind?"

"I'm not sure, what does a pedicure involve?"

"First off, you need to be licensed, or you need to hire someone with a license. Then your shop needs hot water, sinks down near the feet, comfortable chairs, mirrors, and inventory. Once all this is in hand, go to work."

"Clean warm water, soothing the foot. Clean the nails well, remove all the old paint, clip and file, check the heel, it may need sanding, or a pumice stone. Make this entire first-class, Jimmy, it makes the ladies feel like they are getting their money's worth and then some. That's what keeps us coming back, 'we're getting our money's worth, and then some'. Put on a good primer, and do an excellent job painting."

"Jimmy, you'll have a great business; you love to talk, and when the ladies are in the chair, there's nothing better than good conversation."

"What do you get for something like that?"

"Moneywise?

"Ya."

"You do a good job, clip, file, sand, primer and paint, you can charge forty to sixty dollars an hour, plus, there's tip money. Sounds good doesn't it, well it is good my friend, puts you up there with the High Priest.

"How about that date, Rosalie, I'm going to a leather seminar at Donny Johns, next Thursday morning at nine. It will be over by noon, it's just around the corner from you. Why don't I stop by around noon, I'll buy you lunch, and we'll get caught up on old times."

"I'll put it in my calendar, be looking forward to seeing you, Jimmy, and finding out how your pedicure business is progressing."

"Great, see you then, and thanks for the info, Rosalie."

It was six o'clock in the evening when that conversation ended. Jimmy closed and locked The Cobbler Shop, walked down to the Shamrock Room, took his customary seat at the bar, ordered a Bud, and said to Carman Fish, "**I'M IN!**"

Stella and Johnny had been on board the tramper for eight months, scraping, sanding, oiling, painting, polishing, and doing the bright work. All the staterooms were clean, new bedding, shower curtains, and webbing installed. All the lights had new bulbs, and all the latches on the portholes were functioning properly.

Cleats were in place and fastened securely, all frayed mooring lines were discarded, and new lines were in their place. The safety lines around the deck were checked and rechecked for strength, durability, loose screws, and loose bolts. The masts, booms, and pulleys were all worked over as was the crow's nest.

The kitchen was cleaned and polished, new pots and pans, silverware, plastic plates, cups, and saucers were in place. When the rest of the crew comes on board they would be given quarters and fitted with life jackets and survival suits.

Stella and Johnny had their downtime. In the evening, they would stroll down to the 'Big Board' and look for crewmates. They needed a navigator, a shipwright, and a diesel mechanic. A cook and a deckhand would also be added. Through the course of the past few days, they came up with eleven names to choose from. Tomorrow they would begin making phone calls and setting up interviews, tonight it would be steak, tossed green salad, French bread, and wine at Etta's.

"Hi, you're on 'Fitness for the Day' with Johnny Tucson; how can I help you?"

"Hi, Johnny, my name Betty Sue, I live here in San St. Rosalina. I would like to ask how much weight a person should lose in a month? My trainer says she is looking for me to lose six to eight pounds every thirty days. That doesn't seem like very much to me, what do you think?"

"That's a good marker, Betty Sue. If you lose eight pounds a month in ninety days, you've lost twenty-four pounds, how bad can that be? Plus, it means you're not gaining weight, and you are not showing that yo-yo effect of up-down, up-down, every time you step on the scale. It also means you're are eating smart, you're learning new and improved methods of eating as well making a better selection on your food choices.

"Go for it, Betty Sue, listen to her, if you're not smiling today you'll be smiling in three months, I guarantee it."

"Two pounds a week, that's a delight in my book."

Duane Mann was welcomed aboard as the ship's carpenter. He has 30-years of boat building experience and once rowed from Seattle, Washington to Ketchikan, Alaska, in a thirty-foot sea dory he built in his back yard. Duane had all the necessary equipment and at six feet four inches tall and two hundred and forty-five pounds he could double as security guard. He was well qualified and had been blue-collar all his life; he passed the look, feel, and listen test with flying colors. Duane's wife, Ericka, would come on board as the Galley Chef. They had a family of six with grandkids and all; Ericka was well prepared in culinary arts.

It would be a big responsibility for Erica. Sometimes they would be at sea for ten or twelve days at a time. This meant they had to have enough food, especially fruit, to sustain a crew of seven with a minimum of three thousand calories a day. They also had to be plenty of fresh drinking water; this meant the desalination unit had to be functional all the time, the freshwater holding tank only stored twelve gallons. The ice machine had to be working twenty-four-seven. There would also be room onboard the boat for three fare-paying passengers, which meant additional meals and water.

Every port where they docked, Ericka would need to fetch supplies. She would be tramping through open-air markets where she might find fresh fruits and vegetables. Beef, seafood, chicken, and pork would be on the ice; commodities like wheat, grain, and flour would also be needed. Spices, herbs, coffee, tea, and milk would also have to be located and purchased. Ericka would have to hunt, peck, and forge, the budget would be tight.

Vanessa Valdez came aboard as the navigator and the electronics technician. Vanessa had spent six years in the United States Navy learning her trade. After being honorably discharged, she used her GI Bill to attend college at Long Beach State University, where she graduated with a Degree in Electrical Engineering. From Long Beach State, she traveled to Boston to attend M.I.T. After receiving her Master's Degree, she went to work for AT&T, where she would spend the next twenty-two years of her life. Vanessa was bored with retirement and looking for adventure, hiring Vanessa was a no-brainer.

Vanessa began her adult life working on navy destroyers. While doing so she purchased a twenty-one-foot Boston Whaler and from there she jumped to sailing a twenty-four-foot Hoagie Cat, from there it was on to ocean-going kayaks. Vanessa was well versed in life on the water; she could ocean swim three miles with no problem, river swim, scuba dive, and hold her head underwater for a full sixty seconds. On top of all this, she was friendly, personable, and an electronics expert; they couldn't have asked for a more qualified person.

John Jackson was another blue-collar man. He was welcomed aboard as the diesel mechanic/engineer. John was forty-three years old and had been into motors since birth. Throw out a thousand used motor parts, nuts and bolts, washers, a few wrenches and screwdrivers, and John could build you a engine, gas, diesel, steam, you name it, John was born an engineer.

John had a Mechanical Engineering Degree from the University of California, and that was all he needed, John was a field man, not a desk jock. He had driven dragsters, funny cars, and was a pitman at Indy. John had done offshore boat racing and was the captain of a crab boat in the Bering Sea three years running. John looked at the Detroit Diesel engine in the tramper and immediately named it, "Honey."

Sammy Patrone was a traveler. Sammy held a card in the International Brotherhood of Electrical Workers and has spent the last twenty-two months traveling across the continent in his Volkswagen bus. Working here and there, Sammy was visiting family and friends, camping, fishing, swimming, and wondering what to do next.

Sammy posted an ad on the Big Board that read, "Looking for work, an electrician by trade, strong back, strong arms, clear head, drug-free, and willing to travel. If you're looking for such a person, call Sammy…." Stella made the call.

There you have it, the crew was set; seven strangers about to partake in a life-changing event **'COME ON ALONG.'**

Cameron Blue figured he had maybe four, five, or six years left to live if he didn't get a kidney transplant. He was looking at a three hundred thousand dollar bill for the transplant operation with no way of obtaining the money. He knew he was going to die without the operation, whether he wanted to die in prison or at home was up to him. When he took his lunch break, he walked down to the Shamrock Room.

"Hi, Carman," Cameron said, as he entered under the twelve-foot high arching doorway that separated the restaurant from the lounge

"Cameron, good to see you, what's going on, can I get you a sandwich or something from the kitchen?"

"Sure, it's lunchtime; I'll have a bowl of chicken soup and a glass of ice tea, maybe a twist of lemon in that tea."

Carman was on his way to the kitchen when he heard the words, 'COUNT ME IN, CARMAN'. Carman stopped dead in his tracts, turned towards Cameron, smiled, saluted, did an about-face, and continued on his way to the kitchen.

The pieces were falling into place, Carman thought. DH Jimmy was in, Mainland Bill and Sharon were in, and now Cameron was in. Carman had a good feeling about Charmain being in, now it was up to Roxanne Rodriquez being in. In fact, if Roxanne wasn't in, there would be no, 'IN!'

"Hi you're on Fitness for the Day with Johnny; how can I help you?"

"Hi Johnny, my name is Marge, I'm calling from San St. Rosalina. I've been listening to your program for quite some time, now I need some advice."

"Fire away, Marge."

"I go to the gym three times a week, yet my blood pressure keeps on rising, and my weight keeps climbing. Something is backward here, Johnny, how can I stop this backslide or whatever the heck it is, what am I doing wrong?"

"Marge, congratulations and welcome to America, you are not alone with this problem. I'll tell you the same thing I tell the others, it's all in the diet. You can go to the fitness center twenty-four hours a day seven days a week, Marge, but if you're not going to change you're eating habits, well, it's up three and back four."

"Nutrition, the food we take in and not just how much we eat, but what we eat is the culprit here, **too much sodium and sugar,** Marge. Like cigarettes, sodium and sugar are the new silent killers of the American people."

"Marge, for example, let's says at breakfast you eat a two-egg omelet with cheese, a slice of toast with butter, a little jam, not much, you're watching the waistline. Now for lunch, you have a tuna sandwich, with a small salad and a little French dressing, again, not much, let's stop right here and talk this over right now."

"Sodium and sugar in the toast, in the cheese, sodium, and sugar in a jam, sodium in the butter, and that's for breakfast. For lunch, sodium and sugar in the sandwich bread, sodium, and sugar in the mayo, if you have a slice of cheese more sodium, French dressing more sodium and sugar."

"We haven't even touched dinner yet, and that is where the greatest amount of sugar and sodium is usually eaten. Do you understand where I'm coming from, Marge, multiply all this sodium and sugar by the day, by the week, by the month, by the year, and it all adds up to high blood pressure, fat, obesity, and one big ugly sickness."

"An hour or so in the gym will not take care of this problem, Marge, especially as you grow older. "Shop the perimeter, veggies, fruits, lettuce, talk to the butcher, more tuna, salmon, and catfish, throw in some chicken. Stay away from the center aisle when you can, you need coffee, tea, olive oil, and whatever, fine, but hang in the perimeter."

"Sodium and sugar in most of the package, canned, and frozen foods we eat, bad for the B/P and the weight.

Hang in there, Marge, baby steps, great question, read the labels."

"Thank you for telling me this, Johnny; you are such a positive influence for me, I'm going to heed your advice."

"I think I'll call you more often, you're free. I go to the shrink, and she wants an arm and leg an hour. I'm way better off after talking to you, both in my physic and in the purse.

"Call every day, Marge, I mean that, let's get that blood pressure under control and the weight down."

"Good-bye, Johnny."

Tonight will mark the fifth time Carman Fish and Roxanne Rodriquez have had dinner together in the past two months. The first time there was no mention of the caper, the second time there was a drop, the third time there was a drop and a top, the fourth time it was exciting but still only make-believe. Tonight it would be a make-believe story that comes true.

"We're going to do it, Roxy!"

"Do what?"

"Cameron, Jimmy, myself, and my two friends from across the Gulf, and maybe Charmain, are going to pull off the robbery; we need your help, Roxy. You won't be involved in the main caper just the hack into Viola's computer, the police will never be able to trace it to you."

"What are you talking about?" Roxy answered, with a curious and mysterious look on her face.

"Robbing the Ruby Rose Hotel the night of the Gala," Carman answered.

"Were you serious? I thought you were just funning around."

"Really, no, it's for real, Roxy, we're all going to be wealthy, free to travel, live where we want, do what we want."

"Sure, like living in prison, doing laundry, cleaning pots and pans, scrubbing toilets, that's not what I want."

"Prison will never happen, listen, when Bill and Sharon came from across the Gulf a few weeks back, they left their address as a house in Lafayette, Louisiana. They stayed in the Lafayette Hotel the night before they came to San St. Rosalina and brought two pillow-cases with Lafayette Hotel laundry stamped on them. Six days before the Gala, Bill and Sharon will be back in town, check into the Ruby Rose Hotel, and make themselves visible."

"They will use the same address as previously. The hack will appear to come from a coffee house in Lafayette, while suspicion will also focus on the house address in that city. Sometimes, while you're on the CEO's computer, leave what is written on these two index cards." Carman slides the two note cards in front of Roxy.

"What is written on these cards will be tall tale evidence the hack came from Louisiana. The clues will not be perfectly clear, but a good police hacker will spot them."

"Very clever, sweetheart," Roxy replied, "but I have two children at home and can't just risk them for this." "How much do you think will be in the safes?"

"I believe a couple of million hands down. The bulk of the jewelry they'll be wearing that night, but the safes will still house plenty. Whatever the haul, we'll share a percent with the fence. He'll probably want half; I'm going to ask for sixty-forty."

"We'll split six ways, Bill and Sharon will take one cut, Jimmy, Cameron, Charmain, you and me. I figure about three hundred thousand each."

"I don't really need the money, Carman, but the idea sounds exciting. Robbing billionaires of their jewelry while they are parting, who would ever think of something like that?"

"Just me,"

"Yes, I believe that."

"All right, Carman, I'll help you out, but if anything goes wrong, you'll have the devil to pay."

"Nothing will go wrong, Roxy."

Time was getting close for the first sea trial run. The crew was accounted for and the boat was in final stages of preparation. Stella and Johnny had gone through everything but the brain work, now it was time for skullduggery.

Johnny worked with Vanessa as she rewired all the electronics. They ran every piece of wire from the instrument to the switches to all the relays and all the way back to the circuit box. The radar was already up and running, but it was also rewired. Next came the depth finder, then the two VHF radios, the GPS was installed, and finally, the ship's intercom was in place.

Johnny and Vanessa wired two new spotlights, one fore, and one aft. Next were the running lights, green on the starboard and red on the port, and finally the anchor lights. All the interior lights and all the exterior walkway lights Stella and Johnny had already completed.

Duane went over everything in the engine compartment with John. They wrote everything down; they had diagrams for every nut, bolt, and gauge. John said he went by sound, rather than the gauges, he listened to the engine; he knew its purr. If something didn't sound right, he would know about it before the gauges.

The hull was found to be in excellent condition during the survey, as was all the underwater mechanical equipment. Duane said the superstructure was fine; he and Sammy worked on the anchor chain and the wench.

Stella was like a kid in the bosun's chair. The masts were cleaned, repaired, and oiled, the same with all the booms. All lights and pulleys were replaced, lines were replaced. The crow's nest was reworked, oiled, varnished, standing tall and looking good, new sails were in place.

Ericka had the desalination unit up and running and producing about ten gallons an hour. This water was to be the crew's drinking and cooking water. Dishwater, shower water, and toilet water would be filtered, but not desalinated. All pumps, hoses, and lines, were in fine working order and sealed tighter than a drum.

Hot water was on-demand and on a timer. Showers were limited to six minutes of hot water, after which it would be a cold shower. Because of this, the men had buzz cuts, and the gals had their hair cut as short as they could stand it. Although the crew knew about the hot water limitations, everyone was to experience it the hard way.

As Stella so gracefully put it, "We're in ship shape, if anything goes wrong, we'll be the first to know."

Next week the crew would be moving into their quarters and fitted for life jackets and survival suits; the first shakedown cruise was just around the corner.

Stella and Johnny had been gradually growing into one another's company. Eight months onboard ship having breakfast, lunch, and dinner together, watching the early morning sunrise, and seeing the evening sunset can change a person's soul.

Sometimes they would sit on the aft deck and eat a quiet breakfast, other times they would have supper on the bow of the boat. It is quiet and peaceful at the marina in the early morning and evening hours. Work shuts down; there is no rush hour traffic; only the sound of the gulls and the ringing of the sailboat bell.

Quite often, Johnny and Stella would stroll down to Etta's and have an early morning breakfast, and watch the cleaning crew come to work.

The cleaning crew would arrive every morning promptly at three-thirty. Two crew members would rope off a section to be cleaned, other crew members would gang up to help them, two or three cleaning salt and pepper shakers, another wiping napkin holder, one or two would be wiping tables and chairs.

When the tables were cleaned, vacuums would come out, thirty minutes later they sprayed the area with a nice fresh mint smell, ropes would come down, and the crew would move on to another section. That is the way it was done until the entire restaurant was cleaned. They saved the arcade games until last.

Pool tables were brushed, new chalk was added, and the balls were wiped. The glass on the pinball machines was wiped clean; the shuffleboards were swept, vacuumed, and resurfaced. On it went until all the TV's were wiped, books put away, hardwood floors mopped, and the kitchen doors cleaned and polished.

There are no interior walls in Etta's. The kitchen is horse-shoe-shaped and surrounded by a nook and high chairs. There is a six-foot-high Plexiglas wall between the nook and the kitchen. Diners can sit at the nook and watch the kitchen crew prepare various foods and do fancy showboating like twirling pizza dough with their fingers, torching certain foods, or cracking two eggs at the same time.

If a diner wants their eggs over, just a flip of the pan will do the job, no spatulas necessary. The kitchen folks were proud of their culinary skills; they had become actors while the diners were the audience, a good fun-loving show. The cleaning crew wiped the entire outside area, all the Plexiglas, shakers, counter, stools, and menus.

At the far end of the kitchen stood the coolers and freezer, sixty feet beyond them nestled in one area of the building was a two-step elevated platform. This platform measured forty feet by thirty feet and was sectioned off with a four-foot-high partition wall. On the platform were several desks, chairs, couches, and various computer screens. This is where Etta, Big Bill, and several others conducted their business; the crew cleaned this area as well.

"Hi folks, you're on the air with Johnny; for the past several days, I've been talking about Tony Rowland being on the show with us, well that day has arrived, here is Tony (Rock'n) Rowland."

"It's good to have you back, Tony. Let me tell all the fans out there in radio land how outstanding you look; fit as a fiddle' in your Cleveland Indian baseball cap, Etta's T-shirt, Levi's, black Wellington boots and I might add, it looks like you stopped by and had a chat with DH Jimmy."

"Thank you, Johnny, for that grand introduction, and yes I did stop by and had a chat, and a shine, from DH Jimmy. He's such a wonderful person, I always enjoy talking with him, and he does such a great job shinning my boots." "It's hard not to love that guy."

"It's a pleasure being back in San St. Rosalina. The sun is always shining, the sky is blue, the air smells fresh, the Pacific Ocean looks good, and the people are just so friendly, wonderful, and happy all the time. I just love being here."

"Well, we feel the same about you, Tony. How about two gold's and a platinum in one year, how did you manage that?"

"Johnny, as you know, the music business is just like any other business, it takes teamwork. Just like the Green Bay Packers, KETA's, or the Detroit Pistons, it's a team effort from the get-go. In my business there are music writers, lyric writers, backup singers, recording engineers, sound engineers, and production people. If it wasn't for those people there would be no me, they do all the work, I get all the credit. That's how you get two gold's and platinum, Johnny, a good team, and a good team effort."

"I understand where you're coming from, Tony. Let's take this caller and listen to what she has to say."

"Hi, you're on the air with Johnny and Tony."

"Hi, Johnny and Tony, my name is Megan, I live here in town. I would like to ask Tony if he will be playing anywhere in San St. Rosalina during the Gala."

"Yes, Megan, as a matter of fact, I'll be playing at the Monterey this coming Friday night. I will also be playing informally at Etta's throughout the holidays. I'll be in and out of town for the next few days, so if you miss me Friday night catch me at Etta's when you can, Megan."

"Thanks for asking ."

"Tony, you said, informally, at Etta's, what do you mean, informally?"

"I don't have anything scheduled at Etta's, but I'll be coming in from time to time with my guitar, if nobody is on the stage I'm going up and play, morning, noon, night, anytime I can."

"Anyone can come up and join me for a jam session, very informal, no script, no sheet music, just sing, play, talk, laugh, and have fun."

"Richard Day, the owner of the Cleveland Indians baseball team, is going to meet me there Sunday. If there is an empty stage; we're on for a duet, that's about as formal as it's going to get."

"There's always an empty stage at Etta's, Tony." "There are what, three or four stages to play on, always one available."

"Johnny, did I ever tell you how I met Richard Day?"

"No, this should be good."

"Believe me, it is."

"Two years ago, when I was here for the Gala, I went down to the fishing boat as soon as I arrived in town. Richard was on the boat looking around. I said hi, he said hi, we struck up a casual conversation. We didn't talk about anything serious, we didn't even introduce ourselves. As it turned out when we parted, for some reason, and I don't know why, but I thought he was the owner of the fishing boat. Richard was to tell me later that he thought I was the captain of the boat, and would be at the controls during the fishing trip."

"Three hours later, we returned for our charter, and can you imagine the surprised look on our faces when the introductions were made. It was a real icebreaker, a burst of laughter, to say the least. We told the story to the others and we became known as "The Captain and The Skipper." It was such a fun trip; Ton Lu from Japan was on the trip as was Mickey O'Shelly from Ireland and Jimmy Keys, it was just great.

"Six hours of fishing, sunshine, laughter, and I might add a beer or two. Plus, we came back with one hundred pounds of fresh fish." "And check this out; Richard invited me to sing the National Anthem on opening day in Cleveland last season. What a special day that was, not all singers or performers have such a day, a very special occasion, I was so proud, my entire family was there, mom, dad, the in-laws, and the children. A Very heartwarming day, a day that sits on the top of my resume list."

"Richard and I will always be great friends, I love the guy."

"Great story, Tony, how funny! Richard Day, an outstanding gentleman, very down to earth, humble and fun to be around. I met him three years ago at the Gala, and I'm sure he'll be here for this one."

"Congratulations, Tony, on the Anthem, like you said, 'thousands and thousands of performers out there every year but only a few get the call."

"Let's take another call; hi, you're on with Johnny and Tony."

"Hi Johnny and Tony, my name is Jenny, I'm from San St. Rosalina. I would like to ask Tony if he wrote the words to, "I'm Sorry I Never said Good-bye?" I heard that song on the radio and went out and bought the CD right away. It's such a beautiful song."

"No, Jenny, I never wrote the words to that song. A writer by the name of Ella Holland wrote the words, I put the music and tempo to it. Ella dropped the lyrics off with me one day and said, "What can you do with this?"

"That's the platinum Johnny mentioned at the beginning of the program. I'm glad you like it, Jenny, it's a lovely song, and I sincerely enjoyed recording it. Next time I do a live performance, I'll dedicate the song to you."

"Thanks for calling Jenny."

"Let's take a call from Michael. Hi, Michael, you're on the air with Tony Rowland."

"Hi Tony, I would like to know how you balance your career with your personal life. You always seem so happy, honest, sincere, and full of pep. Where does all this come from?"

"Where does all this come from?"

"Good question, Michael, I have to give all the credit to my wife Ginger, and my three children Pepper, Ringo, and Autumn and, of course, the fans. Me, I'm just along for the ride."

"Family wise, we're truly an untraditional family. When I'm home, I'm the one flipping the eggs and pancakes in the morning. I do the dishes, clean the house, and vacuum the carpets, and other household chores. Ginger takes the kids to school, does the shopping, makes sure everyone is at the dentist, doctor, and other appointments, and she keeps the social calendar."

"Pepper is old enough to help out in the kitchen, set the table, bus the table, Ringo and Autumn do what they can, empty the garbage, keep their rooms clean, and look out for one another. We're a real together family."

"When I'm on the road performing, the fans, they truly enhance my life and my performance. I have wonderful graces on both sides of the fence."

"Good question Michael, thanks for calling."

"Hi, you're on with Johnny and Tony."

"Hi Johnny and Tony, my name is Sue, I live in Ocean Beach, I would like to ask Tony if he records videos?"

"I have, several years back when we made "Heart Light and 'Evolution.' To be honest, Sue, it takes a lot of time and coordination to put videos together, and that is the time I would rather spend with my family. My family comes first then my music."

"When I tour, we have live cameras, and some of these recordings are turned into videos. That's about the way we're doing it for now."

"Sue, this is Johnny, good question, and thanks for calling."

"We have time for one more call, Stan, you're on with Tony."

"Hi Tony, I would like to ask you how you stay in such good shape, traveling, touring, performing, rehearsing, and family life, when do you find time to work out. I saw your photo in Rolling Stone Magazine, and you are ripped; how do you do it?"

"Stan, thank you for the compliment, and you're right; it isn't easy. On the bus, I have a small gym, no weights, I use bodyweight; sit-ups, push-ups, jumping Jacks, lunges; and I use balls, bands, and tubes; they work just fine."

"The key is, Stan, to be consistent. When I'm on the road, I go into my road gym and workout for sixty minutes six days a week, no exceptions. When I'm home, I work with my personal trainer, again, no exceptions. I love working out, Stan, I do it for fun."

"That's how he does it, Stan, no exceptions, thanks for Calling."
"We'll be back after this commercial message."

Etta's main job isn't an office job, it is anything but. Aside from hob-knobbing, making the rounds at the restaurant, talking, laughing, and sharing a meal, Etta can be seen watering the flowers, pruning the trees, trimming the arbors, and sweeping the walkway. She lends her name to charitable events; she appears at social functions, sporting events, and is in demand as a public speaker. Etta always has a smile and a warm heart; people gravitate to her, and she feels comfortable in this position.

Charmain Green was cut from the same tree as Etta. She's an, "All American Girl," very crystal clean, smart, with a fascinating smile, and a flair for the dress. Just like Etta, Charmain is a winner and people like being around winners, they gravitate to them."

Carman Fish was also cut from the same tree as Etta; it was no surprise to him when Charmain told Carman she was 'IN'.

"Why was crystal clear and clean, teaming up with a life of crime, Stay Tuned?"

Standing on the dock next to the bow of the boat are Etta, Bill, Johnny, Stella, and the rest of the crew, along with other family members and friends.

Stella steps forward and smashes a bottle of 1942 Mastroberardino Champagne across the bow of the boat and shouts, "I Christen you, the Midnight Rain."

Twenty minutes later, "cast off the stern line," was Johnny's first command, moments later, "cast off the bowline," the Midnight Rain is underway. Twelve thousand dollars and eleven months after Johnny brought the boat to Sunset Bay Marina she was standing tall and looking good as she retraced her steps. She eased her way out of the mooring dock, past the pleasure crafts, the workboats, than through the opening that separates the jetty from the spit, out into Sunset Bay and finally to the blue waters of the Pacific Ocean.

The entire crew is on the deck, or in the wheelhouse; smiles, shouts, handshakes, and hugs were the order of the day. This is to be the Midnight Rains' first shakedown cruise, they were going to go offshore six or eight miles then head north for a few hours, then back to the dock.

All sails are in the wind, the motor was purring, and the Midnight Rain is running smooth. She glides through the water easily at ten, twelve, and fifteen knots. She would hit a maximum speed of eighteen knots.

John Jackson reported to the wheelhouse that everything was functioning smoothly in his corner of the world. The engine was running fine; gauges were working properly, no out of the ordinary noises. John was happy as a clam.

The navigator was checking all instruments and navigational equipment and reported a, 'hearty ho'. GPS was on its mark, radar was functioning properly, both radios were tuned in, one to the coast guard station, the other to the weather station, depth finder was reading two hundred feet, two ten, two fifteen two-twenty, and so on. Vanessa was checking the depth reports with her charts, all was well.

Erica was pleased with what was happening in the kitchen. The ice machine was up and running and would crank out as much ice as they needed. The desalination unit was giving them ten gallons of good clean drinking water an hour and the holding tank was filled to the gallon limit.

Sammy and Duane were checking all the plumbing, water, and drain lines and reporting no leaks in any of the water lines or anywhere in the hull of the boat. The bilge pump was working just fine.

When the Midnight Rain returned to her slip, the crew gathered together for a briefing and detailed report on the happenings; everything was smooth sailing, there were no leaks, no electronic failures, no engine failures, it was a dream come true. Although the crew was looking for a little rough action the waters were somewhat calm, maybe next time on the way to Vancouver, Canada.

In the early morning hours of December 28th, Roxanne Rodriquez was busy in Viola Washington office. Roxy was in the CEO's office for one reason only, to hack into Viola's computer and steal the combinations to the room safes and key cards.

Roxy was a computer genius, but the hack took longer than expected. She was hoping to be out of the hotel and on the road by this time, but she just opened the browser and brought up the combinations. Writing down 114 combinations correctly was something that would take too much precious time, Roxy decided to use the printer. Only one person was at the front desk, and the cleaning crew was vacuuming, Roxy figured the noise from the printer would go undetected. She was right, two pages of freshly printed combinations and key cards rolled out of the printer and not a sound was detected.

Roxy followed the instructions on the two note cards Carman had given her, which would direct the police detectives to a hacker in a coffee house in Lafayette, Louisiana.

When this was complete Roxy hurriedly made sure everything on the desk was in order, shut down the computer, folded the papers and put them in her pocket. Roxy took one last look around, turned off the desk lamp, made her way to the door, made sure it was locked, stepped out into the hallway, closed the door, took off her surgical gloves, and headed for the rear, employees only, exit of the hotel: all went perfect, no noise, not a sound, no nothing.

Roxy was in her car and on her way home, smiling, laughing, and high fiving herself. Roxanne Rodriquez was living the high life, success or death, nothing in between; life on the edge, Roxy's heart was throbbing.

The Gala Dinner kicked off at ten o'clock on New Year's Eve Night. The doors to the grand ballroom were open, and couples began arriving on time. The men were dressed in smart suits, long sleeve shirts, diamond cuff links, and ties with expensive tie tacks.

All wore spit shines from DH Jimmy, diamond rings, and state-of-the-art watches.

The women, of course the night belonged to the women. They were wearing evening gowns galore, red, pink, yellow and blue with necklaces that would stop traffic. They had earrings with hundreds of sparkles and bracelets that would make queens envious. It would be an extravagant night for these ladies; painted toes, painted fingernails, streaks of color in their hair, smiles on their faces, diamonds on their fingers, and pearls around their neck. Tonight is their night, and they are going to ride it to the top of the mountain.

Each round table seated eight and was set with white silk table cloths, the finest white bone china, sterling silver utensils, and crystal drinking glasses. Bottles of the finest Champagne and wines were set at each table. The music was the Eddie Barton Trio, soft, light, and quiet, easy to eat by and tender enough to waltz too.

Two servers tended each table, Prime Rib with scalloped potatoes and a green salad was served. King Crab Legs with melted butter and warm fresh baked rolls were the centerpiece. The wine was poured, water was poured, glasses were filled, and diners were dining.

While the billionaires were partying, the thieves were working, the plan was unfolding...

Carman Fish and his gang of thieves had one hour and thirty minutes to loot 114 safes. Carman and Charmain took their lunch break as planned and made the rendezvoused with DH Jimmy and Gulf Coast Bill at the elevator. Cameron Blue is operating the elevator, he drops Charmain and Bill off on the second floor and Jimmy and Carman off on the third floor.

Each of the thieves carries four items, a master key card to enter the rooms, the combination to all the safes, a penlight and a loot sack. Carman would start at one end of the third floor, Jimmy would start at the opposite end, and they would work towards each other. The same would hold true on the second floor, Charmain would start at one end while Bill would start at the opposite end and they worked towards each other.

The thieves had three minutes to enter each room. They would go directly to the safe, which was always under the right side of the desk, open it, empty the contents of cash and jewelry into a white pillowcase, close the safe door and leave. Remembering, do not to touch anything that was not in the safe. The penlight was the only light to be used, if a room light was on leave it alone.

Four thieves, 114 rooms, twenty-eight rooms each, one hour and thirty minutes to do the job, the timing had to be perfect. Go to the bathroom, fill up on fluids, collect your thoughts, gather your equipment, and stop for nothing. Talk to someone on the head-set if you need assistance, but the action for the night was, 'highball,' all the way.

DH Jimmy carried two extra items; pillow cases, one black, one white. When he was covering the hall security camera, Jimmy carefully concealed his face but purposely let the camera pick up a piece of cloth, but ever so slightly, with a partial imprint of the Lafayette Hotel Laundry on it. Bill would cover the cameras on the second floor, but he would not leave a clue.

At exactly eleven twenty-five, Carman Fish and Charmain Green stopped what they were doing, dropped their loot sacks down the north laundry chute, and proceeded to the elevator where

Cameron picked them up. DH Jimmy would finish looting the remaining rooms on the third floor while Bill did the same on the second floor.

At eleven-thirty, Carman and Charmain were back on their perspective jobs; their meals sat half-eaten in the employee's break room. Carman had Charmain for an alibi, and Charmain had Carman for the same. If anyone should ask, they talked about family life, children, retirement, and the job.

Mabel Huntington, of the Huntington Stables Family down Kentucky way, did leave something in her room. For the first time in six years, someone excused themselves from dinner to go to their room. In the course of the conversation, Mabel was telling Selma Packard, of the automobile family, about her great grandmother's one hundred and fifty-year-old broach.

"I can't believe I left it in the room, it's an etching of my great grandmother, Louise, and she was so beautiful. It has been in the family for four generations, and when I pass, it goes to my daughter, it will be five generations. I never knew Louise, but my grandmother would tell me stories about her; she was such a hoot."

"Maybe tomorrow we could meet for lunch, and you could show me the broach. I would love to see it, it must be gorgeous."

"Well, you know what, we're right by the door. I think I'll tell the door-keep I forgot my pills and would like to go to my room and fetch them. With everyone talking and eating, the waiters moving about, couples dancing, no one will ever notice.

"I'll be right back, Selma."

Mabel excused herself, approached the gentleman standing next to the door, and they both made an exit from the dining room. Mabel was escorted to the elevator, where she was met by Cameron Blue.

"What room number would you like?"

"It's room two nineteen, please."

"Two nineteen, it will be, thank you."

Mabel was thinking out loud to herself, hoping she didn't leave the broach in the safe because she had no idea what the combination was. Frankly, she didn't know if she left the broach in the safe or out of the safe, or where it might be. Mabel was thinking hard, panic was starting to settle in, where is it she questioned herself?

Cameron shutdown the elevator on the second floor turned the lock key and escorted Mabel to her room. When they opened the door the desk lamp was on and there was the broach, right on top of the desk above the safe where she had left it. Mabel sighed relief, smiled to herself, kept her composure, pocketed the broach and casually walked into the bathroom pretending to get some pills. She returned with a big smile on her face, a hug for Cameron, and back to the dining room they went.

"Don't take anything that is not in the safe," were Carman's last words.

It was almost the New Year, Jimmy and Gulf Coast Bill had fifteen minutes to finish up what they could, drop their loot sacks down the laundry chute, and be off the floor at twelve-fifteen.

They did it, finished all the rooms on their prospective floors, dropped their loot sacks down the north laundry chute and met with Cameron. Cameron took Jimmy and Bill down to the basement floor where the hotel laundry room was located.

No one was working in the laundry room; the morning crew would be back on duty at four. Jimmy and Bill exited the elevator through the rear door, hustled down the laundry hallway to the laundry chute and found the bags of loot they dropped as well the bags dropped by Charmain and Carman.

Jimmy untied the knots of two bags, opened them, grabbed several handfuls of cash and jewelry and stuffed them into the second extra pillow case he was carrying, which also had a Lafayette Hotel laundry label on it. He tied all the knots back up, partially hid the Lafayette laundry pillowcase in the laundry cart, and hurried down to the elevator where he and Bill than exited the front door of the elevator and out into the shopping mall.

A little past midnight on New Year's morning, the mall is empty; Jimmy and Bill walk in a tiptoe fashion with urgency in their step as they hug the wall and make their way down to The Cobbler Shop. Jimmy turned off the security system, and in they went, no lights, just the red neon light that proclaimed "closed," and a tiny fifteen-watt desk lamp illuminated their movement.

Into the back room they scamper, penlight in hand. Previously Jimmy had carefully removed a couple panels of the partition wall that separated the store room from the main store. Carefully the bags were placed in the wall, and the wood panels were screwed back in place. Jimmy and Bill hustled back down the hall to the elevator where Cameron met them.

"Good morning and welcome to Fitness for the Day; I'm Johnny Tucson."

"Hi Johnny, my name is Tammy, I'm calling from National City, I would like to ask you a question concerning nutrition."

"I know breakfast is the most important meal of the day, but what does a person do when they are tired of the same old breakfast every day? I've been eating yogurt and peaches, yogurt with bananas, oatmeal with blueberries, and on it goes. A person gets three hundred and sixty-five breakfasts a year, what are we to do, eggs and bacon, toast and jam, cold cereal, the dullness goes on and on."

"Hah, hah, great question, Tammy, three hundred and sixty-five breakfasts's a year; multiply that by your age, and that's a whole lot of breakfasts, and you still have many more to come. You better make the rest of them tasty and sweet with something you love to eat."

"Tell you what I do, Tammy, I improvise. I create my own receipt; for example, I love hotcakes, so first off I blend some buckwheat hotcake mix according to the directions on the box, and then I pour the mix into a glass pie dish and put the dish in the microwave for a few minutes. While the mix is in the microwave doing its thing, I smash one ripe banana with a fork, really pulverize it, and turn it into a paste."

"In the blender, I blend up some fresh pineapple, add a few strawberries, drop in some blueberries or whatever. To this I add a quarter cup of canned peaches with light syrup; this gives the mix enough liquid and the right amount of texture. When the pancake mix is ready, I spread the banana paste on, which replaces the butter

I used in the past. I then pour on the blend, which replaces syrup, and presto, dab is now fab!"

"On the recipe, I jot down how many calories are in the mix, the grams of protein, the grams of fat, the grams of carbohydrates the mega grams of sodium, as well as the amount of sugar. I give the recipe a name and a number, the BK Special No. 6.

"I do the same for lunch, and dinner, this helps keep my weight controlled, my blood pressure down, and I eat what I like."

"Also, Tammy, while breakfast is the most important meal, dinner is the least important. Never load up on food at night, and call it, 'a day', if you know what I mean."

"Thanks for the information Johnny, I can see it's a big effort to do, but over a period of time it would be well worth it."

"You're right, Tammy; it is an effort, my receipts go back nine years, but as you say, over time it's well worth it. Thanks for calling; I hope I gave you some good information."

"We have time for one more call, Rachel, from Ocean City."

"Hi Rachel, You're on fitness for the Day with Johnny; How can I help you today?"

"Hi Johnny, I was listening to the previous caller say breakfast is the most important meal, I've heard that hundreds of times in my life, why is that so?"

"Good question Rachael, 'why is breakfast the most important meal of the day?'

"Let's say you quit eating at eight o'clock Tuesday night, you go to bed at ten o'clock that night, and you get out of bed at six o'clock

Wednesday morning. That's ten hours with nothing going into your stomach. Your digestive system is still working while you sleep; food is being processed and moving through the system, good nutrition going in one direction, and the waste is going in another direction. When you wake up your stomach is empty, it is time to start putting nutrition's back into the processing plant, making ready to feed the body for Wednesday's activities."

"Years ago, when cowboys were out on the range, they woke up and had a good hardy breakfast for the long day ahead. At night they would have a plate of food and a cup of coffee, sit around the campfire, play the harmonica and socialize. There was no seconds, thirds, cheesy bread, loaded potato soup, apple pie, or ice cream."

"The jobs were different for the workers of yesteryear. There were more cowhands, farmhands, loggers, railroad workers, construction workers; they were the push and pull people of America, the blue-collar people, the backbone of our early country. They worked off what they ate, not so today; today, its recliners, TV sets, cheesecake, bulging waistlines, and ballooning hips."

"Go easy on the diner, Rachael, salad, soup, and homemade bread, something nice and something light and only one serving. This will help keep the blood pressure down and the weight low."

"Johnny, thank you for that good information, it's a piece of advice we all know, but never pay much attention to until it's too late."

"Thanks again, Johnny."

"You're welcome, Rachael, thanks for calling."

We all know people with guns and bullets kill other people, and often times themselves; we're always looking for ways to prevent this from happening.

We all know drivers with alcohol and cars kill other people and often times themselves. We know how to prevent this from happening, simply, **NOT DRINKING AND DRIVING**. If we follow this ONE SIMPLE RULE, we can save thirty to fifty thousand lives per year, that's a lot of lives and a very simple rule.

"Play it safe folks **no drinking and driving.**"

The Midnight Rain was scheduled for its second shakedown cruise traveling from its home port to Vancouver, Canada. At fourteen miles per hour, and with about two thousand miles to travel the crew would spend approximately eight to twelve days at sea. This will be a good opportunity to test the crew's nautical skills as well as work out the kinks in the boat.

All the crew except for Sammy, were veteran at sea, they had spent many days on the rolling waters, but none-the-less there were plenty of seasick pills on board. Cast-off was scheduled for ten o'clock on the morning of December twenty-first. Sure enough and true to his word, Johnny was yelling, "cast off the stern line," at ten zero two.

The Midnight Rain was on the move again, past the mooring docks, beyond the breakwater and out into the blue water.

It's a new winter morning in San St. Rosalina. The sea is calm, the sky is blue, and the sun is yellow, but the crew knows these elements will change as they head north into the darker, colder, winter waters of the Pacific Northwest.

Ericka had provisions for two weeks; the crew had full stomachs when they left port, so there would be no lunch on board the Midnight Rain today. The first meal prepared at sea will be dinner between five and six o'clock in the evening.

Breakfast will be served between seven and eight each morning with lunch from noon until one o'clock. Other than those times, the kitchen was off-limits to all but Ericka and Sammy. Sandwiches and fruit could be picked up in the small refrigerator located in the lounge. Coffee was always on.

There were no hitchhikers on board, but the boat did have room for three fare-paying passengers. This meant there could be ten people on board at any given time; the kitchen had to have rules. Erica would be busy cooking, baking, and cleaning much of the day, she needed space.

Course was set; the Midnight Rain turned north twenty-eight degrees from its heading and was northbound to Vancouver.

The boat was now in international waters; she was registered in the United States and flew the stars and stripes. The crew's passports were current, and all the paper work was in order, soon the boat would be in Canadian waters.

At five o'clock in the evening and one hundred miles from home, it was quiet on the western horizon as the Midnight Rain sailed onward. The sky was turning a darker blue, and the sun was setting orange. All exterior lights on board were lit up, the mooring lights and the running lights were on twenty-four seven. It is a quiet and peaceful evening.

It had been seven hours since the gang had breakfast at the Dock Side Café and Ericka knew she had a pack of hungry workers on her hands, the first meal was up. Meatloaf garnished with herbs, spices, and red tomato sauce alongside roasted potatoes with butter and chives was prepared. Freshly baked rolls were on the table, milk, coffee, tea, and water were available. The only request from the kitchen was, "save room for fresh-baked blueberry pie."

The meal was served buffet style, there was plenty for all, and leftovers went back into the cooler to become available for the 'kitchen sink meal' in two or three days.

Ericka kept law and order with the trash; all garbage went into one pile to feed sea life, the burnables were prepared to be burned, and bottles and cans had their place. Erica made sure there were very few bottles and cans on board: why haul it if you can't burn it or feed it to the sea.

Stella, Vanessa, and Johnny would split helm duty, six hours on twelve off. There would always be two people in the wheelhouse during the dark hours.

Eleven minutes after one o'clock on New Year's morning the first call came to the front desk at the Ruby Rose Hotel. At one fifteen, a second call came into the front desk.

Paula Anderson, a twenty-year-old college student, and the part-time desk clerk was staffing the desk by herself. Paula notified the assistant manager of the first call, but the assistant was in a hob-knobbing spirit with the partiers and did not pick up the message. Cameron Blue was running the elevator shuffling the thieves between floors two, three, and the basement, and was nowhere to be found.

In a frozen and fearful state of mind, Paula manages to call 911 after the second call came in. Soon, word began spreading, and spreading faster; the banquet room was emptying, partygoers were on the move scampering back to their hotel rooms. The stairway exits were now unlocked and flooded with people. Cameron had dropped the thieves off and was pushing the up and down elevator button constantly; fear swept through the hotel like a raging river.

"We've been robbed," "the safes are empty," shouts and cries were echoing thru hotel hallways and stairwells as the partygoers began making their way to the front desk. Some were drunk, others were even drunker, and some were not so drunk, but the sobering effects of liquor was working maliciously.

People were pushing, eyes were red, speech was slurred, and fists were shaking, liquor breath filled the air; "Someone is going to pay for this dearly," "My family heirlooms are gone," "How could this happen?" and on and on it went.

By one forty-five in the morning, all 114 rooms in the Ruby Rose Hotel were empty and their occupants are standing shoulder to shoulder in the hotel lobby demanding answers. Greg and Kelly Diamond were front and center, looking despondent, fielding questions, shaking their heads, and assuring the guests the hotel had excellent insurance and the culprits would be caught.

The Dutch people were speaking to the Spanish people, the French were speaking to the Russians, the Germans were speaking to the Chinese, and nobody could understand anybody. Chaos abounded, those who weren't speaking to another person were shouting into their cell phones, "What?" "I can't hear you, speak louder, yes, the hotel, no, not me, well yes, me, and the hotel, what, yes, both, who?"

Half a dozen uniform police officers have arrived on the scene and were standing tall at the entrance and exits of the building. Interpreters were being escorted into the hotel by law enforcement officials; insurance investigators were trying to get in but were being held at bay, the fire marshal and his team was on the scene.

"Happy New Year everyone, this is GeeGee Gambino spinning the records on Radio KETA, 1340 on your FM Dial."

CSI units were combing the hotel when Captain J. Dancer, head of the San St. Rosalina robbery detail arrived; it was two-twenty in the morning. The Ruby Rose Hotel was on lockdown, no one was allowed in or out without police permission.

Yellow crime scene tape cordoned off the entire hotel, including the parking lot. Red and blue flashing lights from police cars lit up the area. Television crews from the city's two stations were on the scene, radio reporters and newspaper reporters were arriving, word was out, billionaires themselves make news, now this, it's gigantic.

Forensic police were dusting handrails, hallways, and light switches. Police hackers were going over the hotel's computers. Captain Dancer was in a mobile van looking at security tapes, going back two, three, four days, looking for anything out of the ordinary; then a knock on the van door.

Three hours after Paula Anderson made the 911 call, a police officer enters the mobile van and hands Captain Dancer a pillowcase loaded with jewelry and cash, it had a Lafayette Hotel laundry stamp on it. Many opinions were being offered but nothing was concrete, now this, the cops finally had something concrete.

Captain Dancer smiled, and was given the particulars, "found stuck in the laundry cart, far north corner of the basement, nothing else around, officers still checking." Dancer thought back deep in his mind, questioned himself, 'where had I seen that name, 'Lafayette,' earlier.' Dancer had his men bring up the names of all hotel guests from Lafayette, Louisiana, in the past three weeks; two names surfaced - Billy and Sharon Packer.

The Captain instructed his men to go back two months; Billy and Sharon Packer surfaced one more time. Dancer became suspicious, but then again, was it concrete? The last time the Packers checked in was six days before the robbery; the first time they checked in was thirty days before the robbery. They stayed three nights the first time and only one night the second time. Dancer's detective instincts were working; he asked his men to bring up tapes of the days the Packers checked-in and to look at other tapes the Packers may be visible in; who they socialize with, who they had breakfast with, lunch and dinner.

The security tapes were carefully viewed, Sharon Packer was hard to miss. She was tall, maybe six feet, long blond hair down to the middle of her back, pearly white teeth, and flaming red lips. Billy Packer held his own, handsome, well dressed, short wavy brown hair, the ultimate couple Dancer thought, maybe the late twenties or early thirties.

Dancer ordered photos of the couple and had them faxed to the Lafayette police department along with details of the robbery. Then, instantly, Dancer remembered where he had seen the word, 'Lafayette'. It was ever so slightly and only for a fraction of a second, but none-the-less, Dancer assured himself the words were there.

Dancer ordered the security tape of floor number three, the night of the robbery, brought up. There it was, 'Lafayette', ever so fleeting and ever so slightly on a black something or other as one of the thieves was covering the security camera. It was only a smidgen of a second, but it was there. Dancer ordered someone to go check that camera to see if it was still covered, it wasn't.

Dancer was sure someone from Lafayette, Louisiana, was in on the robbery. The cash found in the pillow case in the laundry room totaled six thousand dollars; no one would leave that kind of loot behind Dancer thought. And then there was the jewelry, the robbery was too well planned; they must have misplaced the pillow case. And the Packers, from the same city - Dancer was putting two and two together and coming up with four. He had something, and it was all concrete, J Dancer smiled again.

Television crews and reporters from all over the world were now converging on San St. Rosalina. The United States is not the only country with billionaires. Of the 114 suites, only thirty were occupied by Americans.

Hotel rooms in the city we're booking fast. Mexico was already on the scene, Canada was there as well, England, France, Spain were in the air, while Brazil and Argentina were heading north. Japan, New Zealand, Hong Kong, you name it; they were all in the air on the way to San St Rosalina.

Onlookers were showing up along the water's edge, boaters were trolling the spit. Police barricades were still in place: nobody could get in the Ruby Rose Hotel, nobody could get out; the world was outside, the billionaires were inside.

The Midnight Rain was now moving southbound at ten knots from Vancouver to her homeport in San St. Rosalina. The north-bound shakedown cruise had been a success. After a day of resup-plying, minor repairs, sightseeing, and learning the ins and outs of customs and immigration, the crew was once again out in the blue water.

Five hours after setting sail the crew hits a light chop; head-winds are out of the southwest, the Midnight Rain is traveling smoothly. Vanessa is at the helm, the GPS positions the boat posi-tioned sixty-six nautical miles off the Washington coast and one hundred twenty miles south of Seattle. Lunch is up, tomato and tuna salad sandwiches with chicken soup and crackers, coffee, tea, or milk; all is fine onboard the Midnight Rain.

In a few days the crew would be back in San St. Rosalina. After fifteen years on the job at Radio KETA, February twenty-first would be Johnny Tucson's last day. The first day of March the crew would embark on the world tour.

Charts are on the table, Hawaii, The Philippines, Japan, Hong Kong, ports in-between, and ports beyond here we come. Tentative ports of call were pinned on the charts; routs were highlighted in red, fuel depots were marked in green. Plans and preparations had been made; the unexpected would become expected. Connections had been made and were still being made with every organization throughout the world that offers advice and assistance for world travelers.

Stella contacted people she had stayed in touch with throughout the years, Vanessa did the same. Over the past few months, the crew had been depositing small amounts of money into the bank account. The checkbook, which included on boarding fees, registered $11,800, how far that would take them was anyone's guess.

A new adventure in life was about to take hold of the crew onboard the Midnight Rain.

"Good morning and welcome to Fitness for the Day: I'm GeeGee Gambino filling in for Johnny; how may I help you?"

"Good morning, GeeGee, my name is Clair; I'm calling from Fog Point. I'm 67 and have been working out since I retired at age 65."

"Recently I notice my shoulders are rounding and being pulled forward. My mother lives in a retirement home, and when I visit her

I notice all the older adults have this rounded shoulder almost hunch back posture. I don't want that, what can be done to prevent this?"

"Yes, I see that same thing all the time as well, Clair, even in younger adults."

"To prevent this from happening, work your back muscles three times as often as you work your chest muscles. In fact, stretch the chest muscles three or four times a day. Then work those rear deltoids, traps, and rhomboid muscles hard, and lay off the bench press and the peck flies."

"That's the best chance you have for staying square, gravity wants to take everything down, it plays a role, do your best, Clair."

"Thanks for calling. A very important question, stretch those chest muscles, strengthen the back muscles." "Stay Square."

The weather channel is broadcasting small craft advisory off the coast of Washington and Oregon and to stay the distance from the Columbia River Bar, a light drizzle begins to fall.

After lunch, Johnny steps out the port door and feels the chill of the northwest winter. A heavy breeze pushes hard against his chest. It had been years since Johnny had experienced a hard winter, he could hardly remember the cold biting chill of December, January, February, and March, but he felt it today and it was not good.

As the Midnight Rain travels south light drizzle becomes a rain, the wind, which was twenty-five knots, has picked up to thirty knots. The Midnight Rain is rocking and rolling but holding a steady pace. Johnny carefully and meticulously works his way around the boat; he makes sure everything is battened down tight, no loose knots, no faulty rigging. Duane and Sammy are bringing in the sails.

Two hours later, six to eight-foot waves began breaking over the bow of the yawl. The weather channel ups the forecast to gale force winds out of the southwest, increasing to fifty knots; again, small craft advisers are issued. The rain is now a downpour, the lights of the Midnight Rain began to flicker. This is not good.

John Jackson makes a call to the wheelhouse."We have water leaking into the engine compartment." "The main generator is getting drenched; it's shorting out, I'm switching to the backup. If we lose power, it will only be for a few seconds."

"We were hoping for stormy weather, but not this."

"Roger that, John, we are going to navigate closer to the coastline. In the event of an emergency Johnny feels it's better to be thirty or forty miles off the coast rather than sixty or eighty."

"Roger that, I agree, be sure to stay well away from the Columbia River Bar."

"Will do, keep the power on and the engine running, we should be able to navigate through this."

"Are the sails still in the wind?"

"No, Duane and Sammy lowered them, we're solely on engine power."

Waves are breaking over the stern in such a way the Midnight Rain is almost swamped when she goes deep in the trough.

Thirty minutes after the first call to the wheelhouse, John makes a second call, all power onboard the Midnight Rain fails; the second call never gets home.

Johnny sends Vanessa to go talk with John, "if power is lost, bring everyone to the wheelhouse and start putting on your survival suits."

The Midnight Rain was pitching high and low as the waves were dipping and cresting at forty to fifty feet. Water was pouring into the boat from all directions, the stern was taking a horrible shellacking, and the bow was broaching uncontrollably. There was no power at all, all communications were lost, no radar, no VHF no GPS, no ships intercom, no lights, no back-up generator, no nothing, everything was out and the sky was gray and getting darker.

If the crew has to abandon ship, they better do it before the boat capsizes or gets swamped. The Midnight Rain is at the mercy of the wind, the waves, and her own will power.

By noon on New Year's Day, the police had interviewed the hotel employees, the billionaires, and the catering crew; everyone was now free to leave.

Outside the hotel television crews, camera people, news reporters, and onlookers were now gathered by the hundreds. Barricades with yellow barrier tape were still in place; black and white police cars still surround the area, red, blue, and yellow lights flashing.

News helicopters are hovering low in the sky when billionaire Sarah Sue Cross and her husband Tom ducked under the yellow tape and out into the streets of freedom and into the eyes, mouths, cameras, and microphones of the waiting reporters.

Sarah Sue Cross didn't make her billions by being stupid; she was in the public relations business and looked at this as an opportunity to enhance her reputation. Rather than coming across irate, upset, and angry, Sarah Sue faced the cameras with a soft smile, wide eyes, and a pleasant voice.

"What a way to ring in the New Year people, yes, the Ruby Rose Hotel was robbed." Sarah Sue says to the reporters, who had gradually closed the circle around her from yards to inches.

"The people who perpetrated this must have worked for weeks, maybe even months planning it. The police are not going to solve the case in minutes, hours, and possibly even days, but it will unfurl, and the guilty parties will be caught. I have all the confidence in the world in the San St. Rosalina Police Department, justice will prevail here.

Thank you; that is all I have to say at this time, Happy New Year everyone."

Every television set inside the hotel was turned on; the other billionaires saw how Sarah Sue conducted herself and thought the better of it. This was the world looking at them, not just America, look smart, be smart, let the world know you are not a horse's ass. The monetary loss was just a drop in the bucket, 'put your best foot forward,' became billionaire's mantra.

Peggy Hildebrand stood her ground, watery-eyed, and with a quivering voice, she spoke of losing family heirlooms while holding true to a mantra.

"We're proudest of the treasures we inherited from our fore-fathers and fore- mothers, the-hand-me-downs-from mothers and fathers to mothers and fathers, then on to daughters and sons. These hand-me-downs keep going from generation to generation; we know our great mother's wore this jewelry next to her heart. We know the men in our family carried the pocket watch, worn shiny and smooth through generations of use, it's tough to lose these heirlooms."

Peggy fights back the tears and her voice stutters as she asks the thieves to keep the money but return the heirlooms. Peggy makes a good showing and conducts herself well.

She wishes everyone a Happy New Year.

With the crowd outside growing larger in numbers, and inside the hotel the billionaires still jamming the lobby, Greg and Kelly Diamond are upstairs in their home on the fourth floor hashing things over.

"We've had a great run for five years, how could something like this happen?"

"Don't worry honey, it will work itself out, it's got to. We're insured, the insurance companies will cover the financial losses. There was no damage to the structure or the rooms, so things are not that bad. We just need to stand tall, keep assurance in ourselves, and do not cave in. This way, it will be easier for us to talk with the guests, the reporters, and everyone else."

"Yes, you're right, Kelly, there are pins and needles coming from all directions, questions about security, questions about insurance, and questions about the future; let's be reassuring, honest, and straight forward."

"People still love us, they'll forgive us, and they know our reputation is upstanding. We'll get through this."

Alone, in the quiet confines of their home, the knock on the door startled the Diamonds. Captain J. Dancer is standing at the door when Greg Diamond opens it.

"Captain Dancer, please, come in," Diamond motioned Dancer inside.

"I have some great news for you, Mr. Diamond." "Our mounting evidence leads to a group of people in Lafayette, Louisiana, who we believe may have perpetrated the job. We think they had a hacker using a coffee shop in Lafayette to acquire the combinations and the key cards."

"Before the hack took place they sent a team over here to research the plan. After the research team returned to Louisiana, and immediately after midnight on the twenty-eight of December, the hack was executed. The combinations to the safes and the key card room numbers were stolen online. With hard copies in hand, the team returned to San St. Rosalina to execute the plan."

"We've notified the Lafayette police and faxed photos of two people we feel may have been involved."

"Do you recognize either of these people," Dancer asked, as he showed Diamond photos of the Packers.

"No, can't say I do, of course I'm not here all that much." "Honey, come here and take a look at these photos."

"This is wonderful news, Captain Dancer. Maybe the case will be resolved and the jewelry will be returned intact."

Kelly Diamond was shaking her head in a negatively fashion while quietly answering, no, as to the identity of the couple.

"Well, we don't want to jump to any conclusions, but we do have good leads. I'll be leaving for Lafayette in the morning and should have more information within the next twenty-four hours."

"Thank you, Captain, is there anything we can do from this end?"

"No, just sit tight; this is not the best publicity for San St. Rosalina; if you can repair any damages along those lines that would be great."

As Captain Dancer left Diamond's front door, he mentally began piecing the evidence together while walking to the elevator.

The pillowcase with the Lafayette Hotel stamp on it found in the laundry cart, the pillowcase, or whatever it was, that showed up on the hotel security camera with the word Lafayette visible, both, good piece of evidence. That's the good thing about security cameras Dancer thought, they pick up everything, and can be enlarged, re-run, stopped, brighten, darken, you name it, the cameras do it all.

The police hackers are the best in the business; they believe the hack into the CEO's computer came from a coffee shop in Lafayette, another crucial piece of evidence.

Finally, the Packers, what more could I ask for Dancer thought. All this was circumstantial in the beginning, but by the time everything is added together, it's concrete.

The investigation is in high gear, good evidence and concrete leads, great news for the police chief, the billionaires, and the press. Dancer smiled to himself.

The commotion was still abounding when Dancer exited the elevator at the lobby. Hotel personal were changing shifts, employees were coming in and employees were going out. Insurance investigators were on the snoop, interpreters, billionaires, and just about everyone was pushing and shoving, barking, and grabbing. J Dancer was glad to step outside, get some fresh air, some elbow room, and some sort of resemblance of peace and quiet.

It was resemblance in fact only; there was fresh air, but peace and quiet were a long way from the Ruby Rose Hotel.

It was now well past noon on New Year's Day, Dancer had been on this scene since early morning. The fog had lifted, the seagulls were quiet and Dancer was feeling the effects of an all-nighter. It was best to go home and get some shuteye before leaving for Lafayette.

"Good morning and welcome to Fitness for the Day, I'm GeeGee Gambino filling in for Johnny Tucson, how can I help you?"

"Hi GeeGee, my name is Rose I live in San St. Rosalina. I would like to know how to use the mirrors?"

"Sure, Rose, I can tell you how to use the mirrors. I've never been asked that question before, but let's give it a try."

"Stand in front of the mirror with your best posture, Rose, head up, chest out, shoulders back, and core engaged. Wear as little clothing as possible, sports bra, body shirt, shorts, socks, and shoes, no long pants or long sleeve shirts."

"You are at attention in front of the mirror, this is your position. Make all your moves from this position and return to this position. Keep square, don't slouch. With the little clothing you are wearing, you can see your muscles working. You can see the biceps curl and ball up, you can see the triceps extend and stretch. You can see the quads flex and relax, and you'll see the pecks enlarge and return when doing the fly."

"By looking into the mirror, you can visually see your muscles working. If you're all bundled up with clothes, you cannot see this happening. The mirrors are not in place for you to check your hairdo; they are there for you to watch your muscles."

"Always keep your posture square, straight, tall, and rigid, the mirrors will help you do this. They will also help you develop a feel for your muscles; strength training is a visual as well as a feeling. See your muscles work their way through the exercises, then when you become more experience you can feel your way through the exercises."

"Excellent question, Rose, thanks for calling."

Three days after the robbery, everything at the Ruby Rose Hotel was back to normal. The hotel was booking rooms, and the mall was hustling with retail shoppers looking for yearend bargains. The merchants are busy changing storefront windows to Valentine's Day displays.

Captain J. Dancer is in Lafayette, Louisiana, working up a fireball.

When J Dancer arrived in Lafayette, he was met at the airport by Detective Elizabeth Gerry. Detective Gerry has been heading up the case in Lafayette since the San St. Rosalina Police Department faxed photos of the Packers, along with information pointing fingers at a gang from that city as chief suspects.

Gerry drove Dancer to the coffee house believed to be the place where the hack into Viola Washington's computer took place. Photos of Billy and Sharon Packer were identified by clerks as people who had been seen recently in the coffee house. The police had not been able to identify the specific computer, but that part of the investigation was ongoing. New computers were in the coffee house, old computers were at the police station.

From the coffee shop, Dancer had Detective Gerry drop him off at the hotel where he would be staying. He asked Gerry to pick him up two hours later and to bring with her another detective who was to drive a rental car, preferably a mid-size.

When Detective Gerry arrived back at the hotel two hours later, Dancer laid out his plan.

He would take the rental car and drive to the address the Packers used on their registration at the Ruby Rose Hotel. He would park in front of the house and go to the door, posing as a gentleman looking into his family ancestry. While at the door, he would survey the house. Detective Gerry and the other detective were to stake out the house from a parking spot two blocks away.

Dancer was greeted at the front door by a man in his early thirties, stubble beard, and wrinkled clothing, maybe about six feet tall, with short brown hair.

"Good morning sir, my name is Greg Hall; I'm from Los Angeles and would like to inquire about a gentleman named Paul George and a lady named Hillary Hall."

"Do either of these people live here or have they lived here," Dancer asked, as he handed the man two factious photos. "I'm doing an ancestry of my family tree, and it has led me to a dead-end at this address."

"My daughter goes to college here at the U, so while I'm visiting her I thought I would check this matter out in person. The photos are old, but they might be of some help."

Dancer's detective senses were on high alert. Suitcases piled on both sides of the hallway leading to the front door. The smell of burgers cooking coming from the kitchen, a short blond lady move in and out of view quickly, voices heard inside the house.

"No, I don't recognize either of them. Our family has lived here for decades; my grandparents lived here; my dad still lives here. Sorry, I can't help you."

"Lunch, is ready," came a voice from the far-left corner of the house.

"I see, well, that was simple enough." Dancer said, as he retrieved the photos, his detective senses still on high alert. Two cars parked to the left of the house in the driveway, more commotion from other rooms inside the house, living room to the left of the hallway, kitchen behind the living room.

"Thank you so much for your time. I'm sorry; I hope I didn't inconvenience you."

"No, not at all, good luck," the man said as he closed the door.

Dancer called Detective Gerry on his cell phone shortly after he was out of sight of the house and instructed her to remain on a stakeout. Gerry, in turn, tells Dancer that suitcases are being loaded into one of the two cars parked in the driveway. She also says another car pulls to a stop in front of the house and a man and woman exit that car and are entering the home.

Captain J Dancer drives to the Lafayette Police Station and asks Commander Robert Luna of the SWAT TEAM to suit up.

Time marched on.

It is early winter in Lafayette, Louisiana, at six-thirty in the evening the sky is black. A lonely street lamp dimly lights up the neighborhood as the SWAT TEAM moves into position at six-twelve East Beacon Drive. Detective Elizabeth Gerry and her sidekick are geared up and go with three members of the SWAT TEAM to the rear door. Captain Dancer and Commander Luna go with the four members of the team to the front door while two members of the team remain outside. At six thirty-five, the command is given, "GO."

The SWAT TEAMS break through the front and back doors simultaneously and storm the house. Laser light on their automatic rifles are piercing the eyes and faces of anyone not holding a weapon. Shouts of, "On the floor," "Hands behind your back," "Rollover," "Shut up," echoed throughout the single-story dwelling; doors are slamming, people are yelling, disruption takes over the quiet and stillness of the early evening.

Police, in full battle regalia, are moving from room to room, yelling, grabbing, strong-arming, and rounding up all the occupants. Finally, the words, "clear," "clear," "clear," fan the air. Moments later, pandemonium is replaced by J Dancer's voice. "Everyone on their feet and in the kitchen." Three minutes of fear seemed like three years of a lifetime to the people face down on the floor.

Eye to eye, nose to nose the SWAT TEAM members assist the people they just terrorized to their feet. Hands cuffed behind their back the suspects are lead into the kitchen, a twelve-year-old blond girl, a thirty-something lady, a thirty-something guy, a sixty-something guy, a sixty-something lady, a sixty-something guy, two people still face down on the kitchen floor, hands cuffed behind their back.

The two members of the SWAT TEAM who stayed outside and ransacked the cars come into the house.

"Nothing in the cars except suitcases filled with summer clothing, toilet items, beachwear, and Coppertone, nothing we would be looking for Captain."

The older couple on the floor are still face down and motionless when Dancer moves over to addressed them. J Dancer leans down and speaks into their ear, "All clear, you can get up now," as he and another TEAM member bent down to help the pair to their feet, but it was all over for them, the coroner's inquest report read: Heart Failure, Died of Fright.

J Dancer had been a twenty-seven year veteran of the San St. Rosalina Police Department with many citations. He had been a decorated MP in the military, but now there is mustard on his face. News of this evening's happening swept across the globe at full throttle. On the heels of the billionaires being robbed, now the lead detective on the case wrongfully causing the deaths of an elderly couple

THE RUBY ROSE HOTEL, ETTA'S AND THE BILLIONAIRES

planning to go on a cruise to Hawaii with their grandchildren and great-grandchild, what next!

In the hearing following this tragic event, when questioned as to why he didn't steak the house for a longer period of time, Dancer explained:

"When I was at the door talking to one of the suspects, I noticed suitcases packed and stacked at the entrance to the door. When I spoke with Detective Gerry on the cell phone shortly after I left the house, she told me the suitcases were being loaded into a car; I thought the suspects were on their way to the airport. My only thought was to get inside the house before they left."

J Dancer is suspended without pay.

Richard Glory, a hotshot product of the Los Angeles Police Department, is brought in immediately to replace Dancer, no time for a "trainee." A hop skip and a jump down the freeway and Lieutenant Glory is in front of the cameras.

"I've known J Dancer for years, he is an excellent officer, this misgiving will not tarnish his record. He goes back thirty years in law enforcement, in the eyes of his peers he is in the front line standing tall and looking good,"

"He left a good legacy on this case, he has leads, good leads, solid leads, and we intend to follow up on these leads and hope to have people behind bars in short order."

"That's all I have to say at this time, thank you."

"Good morning and welcome to Fitness for the Day, you're on the air with GeeGee Gambino filling in for Johnny Tucson." "How can I help you?"

"Hi GeeGee, my name is Alice, I'm calling from Sandy Cove, and I would like to know how a person keeps from getting burned out on exercising. I've been doing this for two years straight now, and frankly, I'm getting tired of it, but I don't want to quit. Have you any suggestions that may help me?"

"Alice, if you are getting tired of what you're doing take a break. Take some time off, let your muscles and mind relax for a month or two, when you come back change your program. Go from strength training or whatever you've been doing to yoga, or cycling or stretching, see what happens. Change health clubs, you'll meet new people, develop new social contacts. Maybe the new club will have different equipment, kettle balls, ropes or ladders.

"If this is not to your liking, go to a fitness seminar once or twice a week. Find out what other people are doing, just stay involved until you're ready to get on with your next choice."

"No matter what, Alice, nutrition is always twenty-four hours a day, seven days a week, three hundred and sixty-five days a year. Taking a break from proper nutrition would be real dangerous, like walking on thin ice. This is most important when burnout sets in, and believes me; burnout sets in on all of us. You cannot have an exercise plan without a nutritional plan, if you stop your exercise plan, you must continue and modify your nutritional plan. A revision may be necessary, but do not give up on the nutrition."

"Alice, become a nutritional chef, a nutritional specialist, write a book, give a speech, but stay involved, many good choices, my friend."

"GeeGee, you're so right, you gave me plenty of choices I never realize I had, thank you so much."

"Thanks for calling, Alice

"Troy from C L E V E L A N D, OHIO, welcome to Fitness for the Day. Did I get that right, Troy, C L E V E L A N D, Ohio?

"Yes, GeeGee, I live in Cleveland, but I'm out here on vacation, soaking up the sunshine and just loving it. We have tons of snow back home, and this is just great."

"How can I help you, Troy?"

"GeeGee, how can I develop better balance? I really need balance exercises in my program. I'm seventeen years old and I can only stand on one leg for three or four seconds. Everyone else in my class stands on one leg for ten or fifteen seconds, some people even longer."

"I'll tell you this Troy, take a class in ballet, make that two or three classes. That's your best bet; you'll stand on one leg for hours. Ballet is best; barring that, strengthen the toes, instep, feet, ankles, legs, gluts, core, and practice, practice, practice. The arms are not that critical, but from the armpits down, work hard."

"God didn't make us stand on one leg, Troy, that's why we have two. Thanks for calling, enjoy the sunshine, and good luck with your balance."

Six days after the robbery of the Ruby Rose Hotel, Carman Fish and DH Jimmy are busy removing paneling from the interior wall of The Cobbler Shop.

In the quiet and dimly lit storeroom, Carman and Jimmy remove the sacks loaded with the jewelry and cash. They separated the cash from the jewelry and replaced the jewelry back into the wall and screw the paneling back in place.

They count the money and carefully place equal amounts of cash into six cowboy boot boxes. They wrap boxes with brown wrapping paper and duct tape, address them to billionaires, then place them onto a hand truck. Later that day, Jimmy will roll the boxes to his van, if anyone should ask; it's a special order.

Total cash for the haul, two hundred and sixty-seven thousand, eight hundred and eighty dollars, all of it in hundreds and twenty's, cash machine money. Forty–seven thousand six hundred dollars and some extra went into each box. One by one, the thieves, except for the Packard's and Roxanne Rodriquez, would arrive at Jimmy's home to pick up a box of cowboy boots.

On Martin Luther King's Day, Carman Fish takes the three-day weekend and two vacation days to go on a trip. He drives a rental car to the San Francisco Airport Hotel.

Carman carried one box of cowboy boots with him as he takes the elevator to the eighth floor and knocks on door number eight-sixty-four. The door opens and Carman steps into the outstretched arms of Sharon Packer.

After hugs and kisses, an exchange of pleasantries, a couple of beers and hob-knobbing with Sharon and Bill Carman hits the road again. He drives to the San Francisco Airport where he books a late-night flight to Miami.

Sunset Sonny stood outside The Cobbler Shop looking in the window. DH Jimmy saw this and walked outside the shop to ask the man if he would like some assistance. Jimmy had no idea who he was talking to.

"Good morning sir, may I help you with something?"

"Maybe, how much do you ask for a shine?"

"Depends on what kind of shine you're looking for. A regular shine takes about fifteen minutes and costs six bucks. A spit shine takes about thirty minutes and costs you sixteen bucks." Oh! Hold on a minute, Jimmy barks, with a surprise look on his face as he is looks down at the gentleman's shoes, "those are boots; they're different! What kind of boots are those anyhow?"

"Alligator skin!"

"Alligator skin, gee, I never seen Alligator skin boots before!"

"I killed the gator myself; rather, my family and I killed the gator. The thing snuck into my backyard and attacked my son and tried to drag him into the swimming pool. We were having a barbeque; I saw what was happening and grabbed the cleaver and took after the gator."

"I gave him a big whack across the bridge of the eyes, he let go of my boy, and I continued to whack him as he was making his way to the pool." "My son jumped in and began swinging the camping ax, my wife came on board and hit the crap out of the gator with a baseball bat, and all hell was breaking loose. The gator was splashing, blood was flying, we were swinging, yelling, and screaming, what a battle."

"Luckily the gator never made it all the way into the pool, he got as far as the top step, and that was that. Things settled down, the gator was dead and lay right there on the step. We had cuts and bruises and the pool was red with the gator's blood. I had to take my boy to the emergency room he had a hairline fracture of the right fibula, along with cuts from the gators teeth, a living horror story."

"That was the only major injury any of us had though, could have been worse. I had the pool drained and cleaned; of course, it ruined our first barbeque of the year. We ended eating Chinese."

"I told my wife, I said, 'By God, honey, I'm going to get myself some good boots out of that gator,' and you're looking at them." "The boots are a custom fit, my wife has a gator skin purse, and my boy has a gator skin belt."

"The entire episode, the boots, belt, purse, medical bills, and pool cleaning, cost me bundle, so I wear the boots proudly."

"Wow, yaw, right, a bundle and a fight, I would wear them proudly too! What a story, how big was the gator?"

"He was six feet seven inches, head to tail, big enough."

"Was there enough left over for a hat?" "Sit down right here and put your boots on those foot pegs, I'll see what I have and we'll go from there."

"Sounds good to me," Sonny replied, as he climbed up on the bench and set his boots on the foot pegs.

"Were you here for the big hoedown?"

"What hoedown?"

"The robbery they had at the hotel a while back, with all the billionaires."

"Oh, yaw, well I wouldn't call it a hoedown, but I was here; wasn't working though, it was New Year's Day. I know all about it, everyone in San St. Rosalina knows all about it. Most everyone in the world knows all about it, I mean the billionaires, come on now, how massive can it get?"

"Yes, billionaires, they certainly top the massive charts." "How much money did the thieves make off with?"

"Don't know that for sure, nobody knows that for sure. Insurance companies, cops, banks, private investigators, whatever, have it all tied up, but if you listen to the grapevine you'll hear anywhere two to six million in cash and jewels."

"Quite a haul, two to six million dollars."

"Ya, and right here in San St Rosalina, a person would think something like that would be reserved for Vegas or New York, but no, right here in downtown San St Rosalina. We're on the map, right here where I work!"

DH Jimmy was checking his inventory for gator shinning material and had no idea Sunset Sonny was a special insurance investigator for the Queens of the Great Brittan Insurance Company. Queens had outstanding claims of well over a million dollars from the caper and was looking to recover what they could.

Sonny already knew the ins and outs of the robbery, from newspapers, magazines, television news, interviews, filed reports, and other material he had access to. Sonny had many variations of the robbery, he knew as much about the robbery as anyone except the robbers. But, like all good investigators, Sonny knew the best way to find an answer was to ask questions, not read reports; this is why Sonny left his home in Florida and came to San St. Rosalina, to ask questions.

"How long have you been you been The Cobbler?"

"Been here doing the same thing, shin'n, mend'n and repair'n since the mall opened six years back. I not only do shoes, I also do purses, handbags, coats, hats, and sometimes a saddle. If it has anything to do with leather I work on it."

"I understand they have an event here every year; billionaires from all over the world come to San St. Rosalina. That must be something, a small town like this and all that wealth coming in."

"Ya, but I tell you what, no matter what people say those rich folks that come here for the Gala are not cheap, there're big tippers. I make a two or three thousand dollars on tips alone in those three days, other merchants do the same. They hand out money like we give out advice."

"Town folks love the Gala; we treat the billionaires with respect and down-home dignity. We're polite, courteous, and friendly, and they like that. Of course, we treat all people the same way, but sometimes there's that, 'little bit of something, extra special,' that goes into the Gala, and that counts big time."

"Yes, I bet it does."

"Tell ya what, I have some Clear Wax I can put on those boots. It's clear, won't change the color, but it will clean, shine, and brighten'em, they'll look real nice. Charge you thirty-six bucks, go all the way top to toe, take about forty minutes, you'll be real proud."

"Sounds good to me, let's do it."

"Are you in town on business, vacation, or what," Jimmy asked, as he opened the tin of Clear Wax and took out a clean rag.

"Well, I'm not here on vacation, but I'd like to be. What a lovely city, nice beaches, golden sunshine, blue sky, not much automobile traffic. I can see why those wealthy folks love to come here every year, smell the fresh air, the rose gardens.

"I'm staying at the Ruby Rose Hotel, when we finish here I'm going to walk down to the docks and buy some fresh shrimp off one of those boats, get some good cheese, and have myself a picnic in the park."

"Where else in America can a person buy shrimp right off the boat and still in the shell?"

Sonny avoided questions of business. He felt it better for snooping if people didn't know he was an insurance investigator. If he had to cough up any information concerning his occupation he would tell people he was in the insurance business, that was usually enough to get the subject changed.

"What's your name?"

"Sunset Sonny, but most people just call me Sonny."

"Sunset Sonny, what kind of name is that, is that you're real name or a nickname?"

"On my birth certificate, I'm Robert Christenson, but I've always been Sunset Sonny, I don't even know Robert Christenson. My wife doesn't know Robert Christensen, and my son doesn't know him either. My mother had my name legally changed when I was two years old."

"I went through grade school as Sunset Sonny, high school, college, the military, everything I sign my name to is Sunset Sonny.

"I've always been Sunset Sonny, always will be."

"Why did they name you Robert Christensen?"

"It was my grandmother, and I'd rather not go into that." "What's your name?"

"DH Jimmy." "If you're wondering what the DH stands for, it's Down Home"

"Well, nice to meet you Down Home Jimmy."

Sonny is a dashing gentleman, standing a shade over six feet tall with long wavy slicked back black hair, and piercing blue eyes. His mother is Italian and Sonny inherited his dark olive skin and Mediterranean good looks from her, but the eyes came from his Scottish father.

His posture was impeccable. The soles of Sonny's boots were worn down evenly all the way around, and his chest is bigger than his waist. His ears, shoulders, hips, knees, and ankles are all in alignment. Sonny has a sunset earring in his ear and a tattoo of a sunset on his right arm. His articulation is excellent, and his manners are impeccable.

By five-forty that afternoon, Sonny was back in his hotel room, looking at the safe.

It's an excellent safe, Sonny thought, for a professional safe-cracker to pick the lock it would five or six minutes in each room, too much time for this job. An inside job ran through his mind, but the San St. Rosalina Police had gone up and down the ladder over this one and nothing became of it.

How on earth could someone or some people rob all these safes in such a short period of time? Maybe there were a dozen thieves, six per floor, seven minutes per room, nine rooms per man, could be done. How would they get on the floors? Come off the roof, ok, but how would they get on the roof, and someone had to leave the patio doors unlocked. Key cards were simple enough to obtain. All this could be messy, more people more leaks, word would get out and there is nothing on the streets.

Many questions came into Sonny's mind and he needed correct answers, guess work does not apply.

It was almost eight o'clock in the evening; Sonny had an evening dinner scheduled with Irish Kate, head of The Ruby Rose Hotel Security.

Carman Fish spent the morning and early afternoon visiting with his mother and father in Miami. Later that afternoon, he drove to the OK Diner in Miami's Little Italy section of town. He hooks up with Franky, the Fence, Racoco, for an early supper.

"Here's the deal, Franky, in this envelope is twelve hundred dollars cash and a phone number." Carman slides a yellow envelope across the table to Franky.

"On January twenty-fifth you fly to San St. Rosalina and check into the Toms Hotel; a room will be reserved for you. Call the number in the envelope after you get settled and I will schedule a time to pick you up."

"We will drive to the location of the jewelry; you can make your appraisal then and there. At dinner that evening you will give me a one-time-only number, no second chances. I will accept or reject your number on the spot. If I accept the number you must wire transfer the money to a bank account in Switzerland, I will give you the number at that time. Once the transaction is complete, I will drive you to the airport where a charter flight will be waiting to fly you and the jewelry back to Miami. If I reject your number I'll drive you to the airport where you will fly back commercial."

Franky Racoco realized what having jewelry from this caper meant, the caper of all capers, and Franky would have the goods. This is unimaginable he thought, but it is real, it is happening, Franky pinched himself. The wealthiest people in the world, and he would have their jewelry, how could he be so fortunate. Franky's mind wondered back in time, he had no idea that buying several thousand dollars in hot items from the "Cat Burglar'" a few years back would lead to this.

After dinner, Franky hurried home to put the pencil to paper. Franky figured he would follow his usual routine, he would examine the jewels, ponder them, write a value down on paper, add the sums, and offer Carman one half of the total. Normally he would offer thirty percent of the total, sometimes he upped it to forty percent, but this was special, Franky wanted these jewel in a bad way and it was a one-time-only number.

In the underworld Franky is known as a middle-class fence, having this jewelry in his hands would push his status into the 'higher upper class' status, the Picasso, the Rembrandts, the Michelangelo's of the fencing world. Big money is in arts, but jewelry of this magnitude would add considerable luster to his name. He and his wife would be invited to the big parties, New York, Paris, Rome, Hong Kong, no more Cleveland, Portland, Detroit, or Omaha, Nebraska.

As in any underworld business word would leak out like it usually does; this is one leak Franky would be looking forward too.

Franky began making phone calls and adding sums.

Three days after his meeting with Carman, Franky called in as many IOU's as he could. On this day he had accrued over four million dollars into his offshore bank account.

This includes money from the IOUs, money from sales he hurriedly accepted cash for, money from his own personal bank accounts, money that was already in the account, and money he borrowed.

Franky figured the billionaires would be wearing the cream of the crop the night of the robbery, but he also figured there would be plenty of good stuff in the safes. He was absolutely sure he would double or triple his investment. What would my number be Franky thought; I will know when the time comes?

On the plane ride back to San St. Rosalina, Carman Fish was thinking of his plan. He did not tell Franky that his offer would be the only offer on the table, let Franky bid against himself was Carman's plan. Carman did not want too many hands in the pot, there were already six, and Franky made seven, which was enough. High or low, Franky's bid would be it, accepted on the spot, no rejection possible.

Carman had no idea what the jewels would fetch, but he figured if each thief could get three hundred thousand from the jewels, it was well worth the risk. Coupled with the forty-forty thousand dollars in cash, that would be heading into the half million dollar range.

"Good morning, you're on "Fitness for the Day" with GeeGee Gambino, how can I help you today?"

"Good morning, GeeGee, my name is Jackson; I live in Quiet Cove. I would like to ask what is meant by the term 'be specific?' I hear it all the time on TV fitness shows, and often I hear the trainers in the gym tell their clients, 'be specific?' "

"Good question, Jackson, 'be specific.' That phrase refers to 'how are you going to obtain your fitness goals?'

"You cannot just say, 'I will lose twenty-five pounds this summer,' and leave it at that and expect to lose twenty-five pounds. 'Be Specific,' means, how are you going to lose those twenty-five pounds this summer?

"You are going to go to the gym every Monday, Wednesday, and Friday and work out for fifty minutes each of those days. You will go for a two-mile walk every Saturday. You will have only one medium plate of good healthy nourishing food at each meal. You will turn your snacks into health and fitness bars, oranges, and raisins, forget the chips, dips, and cookies and coke. You will do this for three months."

"That is how you are going to lose those twenty-five pounds."

"Now, you are 'specific', Jackson, you have defined a specific way; you have a plan, a road map, a working set of blueprints. You're going to the gym, you're going for a walk, and you're going to take the proper course of action with food, and you set a time; you're going to do this for three months, exercise, nutrition and time."

"Do I make myself clear on this, Jackson? It is as if you're going from Quiet Cove to Akron, Ohio, you would follow a road map. Same thing here, you have mapped a course to follow."

"Every time you set a goal, plan a specific course of action on how you are going to achieve that goal." "And be sure to put a time limit on it."

"Thank you, GeeGee, good explanation; I understand completely what you're saying. You are excellent at explaining things."

"Thank you, Jackson, and always remember, set obtainable goals."

All the survival suits were hanging in a quarter berth in the wheelhouse. Each suit had a name on it, Duane, Erica, and Stella put on their suits first.

When Vanessa, Sammy, and John Jackson made it to the wheelhouse, they put on their suits. Johnny Tucson put on his suit while Stella took the wheel. The stern was in the water, and the bow was riding high. Johnny figured the best chance to abandon ship was on the leeward side when the boat was low in the trough and tipping towards the sea. Before the crew left the wheelhouse Johnny yells final instruction.

"Hold on to something solid, unhook the safety lines, stand next to the edge of the boat, DO NOT SLIP OR FALL! When I yell jump, jump, do not hesitate. Jump as far away from the boat as possibly. Swim as fast and as far away from it as you can get. You'll be on your own, the waves, the wind, and the ocean are going to take each of us where they want, do the best you can. Let's get out on the deck."

Outside the wheelhouse, the winds were fierce, and water was everywhere. The boat was pitching and rocking, the footing was tough but the crew made it to the safety lines. They quickly unhooked the lines, Johnny and Stella activated their GPS, seconds later the timing was perfect, Johnny yelled, "JUMP," and seven souls jumped into the rough and tumbling frigid winter waters of the Pacific Ocean.

The GPS transmitted signals to a satellite; this message is transmitted to a Coast Guard Station in Virginia, which immediately transmitted the message to a Coast Guard Station in Astoria, Oregon, five minutes later, helicopters are in the sky.

The water temperature in the Northern Pacific Ocean is about fifty degrees. With their survival suits on the crew had maybe an hour or so before hypothermia began to set in. The crew had to hope the GPS beacons and the satellites were doing their job, and the water, wind, and waves carried them far enough away from the sinking Midnight Rain they would not get caught in the undertow.

Waves were now cresting at sixty to seventy feet, the only thing the crew had in their favor was there was still a bit of daylight left, but the sky was dark and gray and getting darker, rain was pouring down, were the GPS's working?

All the transmissions were doing their job. Forty minutes after the SOS hit the Coast Guard station in Astoria the boat was spotted. Two big helicopters were hovering overhead a hundred feet above the tossing water. Spotlights, floodlight, and flares were lighting up everything.

Communicating with one another, the chopper pilots spotted seven people in the water and a sinking vessel about one hundred feet away. The bow of the vessel was still out of the water allowing the chopper pilots to read the name, "Midnight Rain."

This information was radioed back to the base in Astoria. News reporters monitoring the Coast Guard airwaves picked up this information and began checking the name and registration of the Midnight Rain.

Soon news reports were on the airwaves:

"The Midnight Rain, a seventy-foot pleasure craft registered to Johnny Tucson of San St. Rosalina is sinking in severe winds and heavy seas 50 miles off the coast of Oregon. No reports of who was on board, Coast Guard rescue operations are underway."

Radio station KETA in San St. Rosalina picks this news flash up. Afternoon Disc Jock Tony Wolf makes a phone call.

"Hello?"

"Etta, this is Wolf at the station."

"Yes, Wolf, what is it?"

"I just picked up a news flash off the hotline that Johnny Tucson's boat, Midnight Rain, is sinking off the coast of Oregon."

"What!"

"Yes, Etta, it's correct. The report didn't say anything about who was on board, but it did say the Coast Guard was on the scene, and rescue operations were underway."

"I'll be right over, Wolf. Is this news on the airwaves?"

"Yes."

"Ok, see you shortly."

Etta and Bill were still at the Ruby Rose Hotel, the crowd was massive.

"Bill, that was Wolf on the phone; he just told me Johnny's boat was sinking off the Oregon coast."

"What, what the hell!

"Yes, let's get over to the station right away."

Etta and Bill take the stairs to the main floor; walk through the crowd in the hotel lobby and out the front door of the Ruby Rose Hotel, Etta answers the first question from the reporters.

"Etta, were you in the hotel during the robbery, what about it, Bill?" Microphones are shoved into Etta's and Bill's faces, red T V camera lights come on.

"Yes, we were there, and yes, the hotel was robbed," Etta answered. "But right now we have something more important on our mind, we have a personal emergency."

"Our beloved Johnny Tucson's boat is sinking in severe weather off the coast of Oregon. We are on our way to the radio station at this time to find out additional information."

"Please excuse us; we will answer more questions as we find out more answers. Thank you."

Big Bill takes Etta by the arm and begins moving through the crowd fending off reporters with his free hand. The crowd is stunned, momentary silenced, than questions fill the air,

"Johnny Tucson, what about Johnny Tucson, whose boat is sinking?" Reporters began to disperse, making to their vehicles to pick up news feeds.

Bill and Etta leave the hotel and head towards the flagstone walkway. It's News Year's Day, onlookers are everywhere, at the marina, at the hotel, and in the park. Bill and Etta are sidestepping everyone, eyes transfixed, heads focus straight forward as they hurriedly step onto the flagstone walkway, past the Polish hot dog stand, under the arbors, barely saying a "hello," plenty of, "sorry not now," and "please excuse us we're in a hurry."

Arm in arm, they bypass going through the restaurant and scamper along the outside. A hundred feet down the blacktop walkway that separates the restaurant from the restrooms, they reach the business offices.

Bill unlocks the front door; they hustle inside hurry up the stairs and quick stop short of the glass wall where Wolf is working. The red light, "ON THE AIR," is lit up, Bill and Etta wait, twenty seconds later the light goes off, Wolf motions the couple in.

"I don't know anything new, Etta, Bill, check with Rita she has a call into the Coast Guard Station at the Tubbs Light House, they may know more."

Rita's office is adjacent to DJ's, as Etta and Bill entered, the phone is ringing. Rita lifts the receiver out of the cradle and speaks into it.

"Good afternoon, this is Radio KETA, how may I help you?" Rita pressed the speaker button.

"Good afternoon, this is Seaman Janice Upton from the Coast Guard Station at Tubbs Light House. I have the latest report concerning the Midnight Rain."

"Go ahead, Seaman Upton."

"The Coast Guard Station in Astoria reports there are two helicopters in position at this time. The 'Midnight Rain' is sinking and almost totally submerged. There are survivors, they are in the water. The choppers are fighting gale-force winds with waves cresting at sixty to seventy feet."

"Expert swimmers are also in the water and they have rescued one person, Duane Mann. He's aboard one of the choppers, and they say he appears to be in good health. The entire crew of the 'Midnight Rain' made it into the water. That's all I have at this time."

"Seaman Upton, this is Etta at KETA, do you have an open line to the Coast Guard Station in Astoria?"

"No ma'am, we call them on the telephone."

"Do you call them, or do they call you?"

"We call them, we're concerned about this ourselves ma'am. Not only are we concerned about saving lives but were also concerned about Johnny Tucson, he's one of our own. We'll be on top of this to the end."

"Thank you so much, Seaman Upton, can we call you back?"

"Yes, by all means, but give us thirty or forty minutes. This is a rescue operation, and they are fighting gale-force winds with waves sixty to seventy feet. It will not be easy going and may take hours."

"Yes, I understand, Seaman Upton. Thank you again, and we'll be in touch."

"You're welcome, goodbye, ma'am."

"Rita, if any additional information comes in either over the phone or on the hotline, please notifies me on my cell phone."

"This is a bad start for the New Year, first the hotel, now this. Let's pray they're all still alive and healthy."

"Good-bye, Rita, Happy New Year."

"Good-bye, Etta, Bill, Happy New Year to you as well."

"Hi, I'm GeeGee Gambino filling in for Johnny Tucson, you're on Fitness for the Day, how can I help you?"

"Hi, GeeGee, my name is Lorie; I'm from San St Rosalina. Can you tell me what the trainers mean when they say, body weight, only?"

"Yes Lorie, of course, 'body weight', means just the weight of your body. For example, when you do a chin-up, you pull up only the weight of your body. Same with a push-up, when you do a push-up it's just the weight of your body you are pushing up.

"Chin-ups, push-ups, set-ups, Jumping Jacks, running in place, just to name a few, a person does not use weights with these exercises."

"Thanks for calling, Lorie."

Rita had called Etta twice over the past hour to give her progress reports, Etta's cell phone rings a third time.

"Hello."

"Etta, great news, the Coast Guard has just informed me that all seven crew members of the Midnight Rain have survived. They're all in good health and onboard helicopters on their way to the Astoria Coast Guard Station, how wonderful!"

"Yes, that is excellent news, Rita, now we can celebrate the New Year. Did they say when they would be home?"

"No, but I bet we'll know soon, I'm sure they'll be making phone calls."

"Yes, they would have no reason to stay in Astoria. Tell Wolf to spread the good word, the City of San St. Rosalina knows about this by now, and they're waiting to find out, 'the rest of the story.'"

"You're right about that, Etta; the phone has been ringing off the hook."

"Thanks, Rita, Happy New Year, good-bye."

Etta tells Bill the good news, hugs and kisses were handed out. Champaign is uncorked, and even though it is close to January second, the New Year's Celebration gets under way.

On January twenty-fifth, Franky Racoco arrives in San St. Rosalina. As pre-arranged, he checked into the Toms Hotel and calls Carman Fish. At noon the next day, Franky begins pulling jewelry out of the loot sacks.

He puts his magnifier to his eye and looks thoroughly at the piece. He checks the setting, he checks the color, he checks the sparkle, the clarity, and he checks for scratches. Hand to hand he feels its weight and then he rubs his fingers lightly across the piece to feel its goodness.

After Franky finishes checking the piece he pondered it, thinking to himself, 'What can I do with this piece of jewelry.' 'Can I sell it whole, would I take the jewels out of the setting and sell them separately; was the setting worth melting down, could I combine different stones with different pieces? Where will this piece of jewelry lead me'? After 40 years in the business, Franky had options and connections. He could take a piece of jewelry and totally rearrange the configuration so it wouldn't be recognizable to the owner even though the stones and setting were the same.

When Franky finished pondering the piece he tagged it with a number. On a separate sheet of paper, he wrote that number down, placed a value beside it and made a written notation as to his thoughts about the piece.

Two short breaks and six hours later, Franky had three hundred and forty-seven numbers written down. The haul included earrings, cuff links, bracelets, necklaces, Super Bowl rings, tie tacks, watches, broaches, wedding rings, special occasional rings, rubies, diamonds, sapphires, pearls, a hat pin, a gold tooth, heirlooms, and miscellaneous.

The total weight of the haul was thirty-eight pounds. Neither Carman Fish nor DH Jimmy saw the numbers Franky had written down.

The small back room of The Cobbler Shop had no ventilation, it was hot, sweat was dripping down Franky's overweight body, time to go back to the Toms Hotel and freshen up, dinner would be at eight.

San St. Rosalina is known for its seafood, and seafood is what it is. Franky, Jimmy, and Carman were seated at a table in Etta's Restaurant dining on baked steelhead, mussels, tossed green salad, and sweet potato. Franky slides an envelope across the table to Carman, inside the envelope is a piece of paper with the 3.6 million written on it. Carman nodded his head in approval, the deal was on, Champaign was ordered.

Etta is ushering Sunset Sonny and Irish Kate to a dinner table when Sonny noticed DH Jimmy. Sonny paused slightly at the table, said a brief hello to Jimmy, thanked him again for the shine, nodded to Franky and Carman, and continued following Etta and Kate.

Who is that guy sitting next to Jimmy, Sonny thought, he looks familiar?

The wind keeps on blowing, the tide keeps on rising, and Sunset Sonny keeps on working.

High turnover in the hospitality business is nothing out of the ordinary. Employees come and go at a higher percentage rate in this profession than in other professions, so it wasn't surprising when Cameron Blue left his job.

After five years of running the main elevator at the Ruby Rose Hotel, Cameron had given his notice on Christmas Day, telling folks he would be leaving on the fifth of January. Cameron would be heading north to Seattle to find out what he could about kidney transplants. Seattle had become a hotbed of late in this field and Cameron needed all the information he could get, and this included financing.

The fifth of January had come and gone. There were parties held in Cameron's honor, well-wishers offered him the best and time marched on.

Cameron had thirty-two thousand dollars in his savings account, couple this with his share of the cash from the caper and he over seventy grand, plenty of traveling money.

When the jewels are sold, he would have more money, how much more he didn't know, but high hopes were in the neighborhood of a quarter-million. Cameron needed over three hundred thousand for the kidney transplant alone, and then there would be recovery and much more. Cameron wanted to live; he needed big money in a big way.

Best of luck, Cameron!

While it was no surprise about Cameron leaving, it was a surprise when Charmain Green and Carman Fish sent out wedding invitations to family and friends announcing their upcoming marriage on Valentine's Day.

Charmain and Carman had become an item of late, but no one expected this. After the wedding, the couple will head to Miami and spend time with Carman's parents. From there, the newlyweds will travel to Iowa where Charmain's family lives. The twenty-second of February would be their last day on the job.

'Love at first sight', was the answer as to why crystal clean and clear teamed up with Carman Fish. Charmain fell in love with

Carman the moment she laid eyes on him, "He was the one for me, regardless. I set the bait, the fish was hooked, and the courtship was on." That's the way Charmain put it, but don't tell anyone.

Congratulations to Charmain and Carman.

Sunset Sonny sat down one afternoon to read Roxanne Rodriquez's bio sheet. The reading led him to the name of Elijah Torrez. Elijah was a Brazilian coffee baron whose millions were on their way to becoming billions. His wife died in a single car accident several years back and Elijah was raising their two boys, who are now high school age, as a single father. Although Roxanne dated other men it appeared she and the Brazilian had a good liaison going for a couple years. Most of the Ruby Rose Hotel employees knew of this arrangement but it was definitely a shock, when on a Monday morning Roxy showed up for work with a ring on her finger the size of Mars.

It wasn't an engagement ring, it was a wedding ring, the couple tied the knot at Our Ladies of Lords Church in Mexico City over the weekend. Dinner, drinks, and many small parties were abounding for Roxy for the next several weeks and many days thereafter.

Rosanne had told Viola Washington this event was going to happen several weeks back, but it was on the QT. Viola already had Roxy's replacement in line, a going-away party was scheduled for June sixth, when Roxy's children would be out of school for the summer; the family will be moving to Rio shortly thereafter. Rio will be their home away from home; Elijah has a Lear Jet that will keep the group traveling back and forth to grammas and granddads at their convenience.

Paperwork, Sonny thought, where does a person go in this world without paperwork? Names must be spelled correctly, middle names are needed, dates must be accurate, times must be correct, and the filing must be done and done right. Miles and miles, stacks and stacks of paperwork, pencils and pens, addresses and phone numbers, brothers and sisters, nearest living relative, male, female, black, white, Native American, Hispanic, or other. Descriptions, just the facts ma'am, the who, what, when, where, and why; everybody in the world has paper work on them, some more and some less, are Sonny's final thoughts on this matter.

Where in the hell did Lieutenant Glory get his script, Sonny wondered, "J Dancer has good leads," a horse's ass.

When J. Dancer was relieved of his duties as the lead investigator in the Ruby Rose Hotel caper, the paperwork was totally out of whack. The addresses were wrong, names were spelled incorrectly, and the filings were not updated and totally out of order. Notes were missing, dates were inaccurate, food smears and coffee stains over half of the papers, it was more of a pain in the ass then a real pain in the ass.

Sonny spent six days in San St. Rosalina and Lafayette, Louisiana, just undoing the wrongs of paperwork.

Sonny asked questions, reread newspaper stories, watched old news clips, asked more questions, and dug deep; finally he had all the wrongs righted and all the paper work in order. The end game was, Sonny didn't know what he had, on the seventh day he rested.

Who was that guy sitting with DH Jimmy at Etta's, Sonny wondered?

Sonny put in a call to Irish Kate, and they set a time to meet for lunch.

At twelve forty-five, Sonny walked into the lounge at Shamrock Room and stares hard at Carman Fish. Who is that guy, I should know him, where have I seen him before, Sonny is thinking. Irish Kate arrives and the two take a table by the window looking out onto the courtyard.

"Kate, do you know the bartender?"

"Yes, his name is Carman Fish, why do you ask?"

"He looks like someone I know or someone I should know. Do you have any background on him?"

"No, but I could check his employment file."

"Let's do that after lunch; I'm going batty or stir-crazy thinking I know this person or that person. I saw DH Jimmy the other evening when you and I were going to dinner at Etta's, I thought I knew one of the men Jimmy was dinning with, but I can't place him. It keeps playing in the back of my mind, faces and places with no names."

"Carman Fish was one of the men having dinner with Jimmy. I remember seeing him there, but I didn't know the other gentleman."

"That was Carman Fish having dinner with Jimmy that night! Sure, they would know each other from working here. Who was the third person, let's find out who that third person was, how can we do that, Kate?"

"We could just ask Carman, or Jimmy, I'm acquainted with both."

"No, I was thinking of something a little more subtle. I don't want to spook anyone."

"What! You think Carman and Jimmy may have had something to do with the hotel robbery? They're not part of the hotel, Jimmy works in the mall and Carman works here in the bar. A cobbler and a bartender pulling off the biggest jewel robbery in world history, no, I don't think so!"

"To be honest with you, Kate, I just have to start somewhere. I need to get something going in a forward motion. I've been backed up in paperwork since I've been here, I have to start somewhere; Carman Fish and DH Jimmy are as good a place as any."

"Yes, I understand where you're coming from, I see Kelly Diamond every day and she asks me how the investigation is coming along."

"Kelly Diamond, the owner of all this, I'm standing around singing the same old same old, 'we're still investigating.' I'm tired of saying it, and she tired of hearing it. I need something solid, or I may be given my walking papers."

"I'll agree, Carman and Jimmy are as good a place to start as any."

After lunch Sonny and Kate walked down to the Shamrock Room's office. As Kate is head of security for the hotel, which includes the mall, she was given whatever she requested.

"Carman Fish's previous address was Miami, Florida."

"That's my home town," Sonny said softly, and surprisingly, "that's where I must have seen him, maybe his picture was in the paper."

"I have a friend with the Florida State Highway Patrol; I'll give him a call."

"Ok, I'll check DH Jimmy's finances. I heard he was having a hard time making ends meet. I'll see if there is anything out of the ordinary."

"Hi, you're on Fitness for the Day with Johnny Tucson: how may I help you, Reggie, from High Port?"

"Hi Johnny, welcome back, scary times, huh. I wouldn't want to have been floating around in that cold water in the middle of the winter, or any time of the year."

"Thank you, Reggie, I hear you loud and clear, I wouldn't wish that on anyone. What's on your mind, Reggie?"

"Johnny, I would like to know if strength training will help a person lose weight."

"That's a good question, but it comes with a difficult answer, Reggie. Let's just say it plays a role but not the way you might think."

"A person builds muscles through strength training and muscles require plenty of calories to sustain. Simply put, the harder your body, the more calories you burn just to keep it hard. Burning calories is what weight management is all about. Strength training plays a role in weight management, but not necessary in losing weight; just keep your body hard, Reggie, and you'll be ok."

"Thanks for calling; you might want to talk this over with a nutritionist."

"Look that one up all you folks out there in research land. 'What role does strength training play in balancing the scales?' "Give me a call back here at radio 1340 and explain it to me."

"Hi and welcome to Fitness for the Day, I'm Johnny; how can I help you?"

"Hi Johnny, my name is Karen, I'm from San St. Rosalina. It's good to hear your voice, you're my ten o'clock alarm clock, and I don't want anything to happen to you."

"My son, Tommy, is a sophomore in college, and next year, he must declare his major. He is thinking along the lines of health and fitness but not sure of going into strength training, physical education, sports medicine, or where. Just out of curiosity, what would you recommend?"

"Karen, thanks for the call, it is nice to know I'm your ten o'clock alarm clock and you would feel lost without me."

"**Nutrition**, that's where I would tell Tommy to go, you'll never ever and I mean never regret that decision. Not only for your own health and your family's health, but there is such a demand for nutritionist in this world you would never have to worry about being unemployed. Nutritional education, do we ever need that in the American homes today. At every level in our society, whether be upper class, middle class, or lower class, along with ethics and values, nutrition should be on the family discussion table.

"From the beginning of your life to the end of time, Karen, nutrition is your most important ally. Families split up, husbands and wives come and go, children come and go, injuries come and go, money comes and goes, but nutrition stays with you forever.

"That's where I would tell Tommy to go, Karen**, Nutrition**."

"Thank you so much Johnny, I'll tell Tommy what you said. I bet he'll be surprised! He never mentioned that in his list of choices."

"Thanks again, see you tomorrow at ten, or rather, be listening to you tomorrow at ten, bye."

Audios, Karen.

Sonny's friend, Chief Inspection Dan Topping, returned Sonny's call and over the next few minutes, informed Sonny that Carman Fish had been under suspicion in several insistences.

He was questioned several times and was under surveillance concerning his boat in drug-related activities in the Gulf, nothing became of this.

He was under suspicion again for the 'Cat Burglar' capers, but only because of the Gulf happenings and the fact his high school sports uniform numbers correlated with the floor numbers of the missing jewels, again nothing.

Topping told Sonny about, 'The Pitch,' as well as the fact Carman had stolen a car several weeks before, 'the pitch', but was never charged. "Carman Fish," Topping said, "was too big of a spender for the job he held."

"How could he afford a hundred-thousand-dollar cigarette boat, live in expensive condos, have two high profile marriages with high maintenance wives and two divorces, on a bartender wage?" "He's not even thirty years old; he's getting money from out-side activities."

That was it on Carman Fish, a suspicious character to say the least, but no meat on the bone.

"If you come up with anything, let me know," were Topping's closing remarks.

Carman Fish was under suspicion when unsolved crimes were committed. As far as Sonny was concerned, under suspicion and unsolved crimes are related, they go hand in hand. Sonny was going to continue looking into Carman Fish.

DH Jimmy's financial report was accurate for the past five years, except for a few weeks ago. Irish Kate found paperwork attesting to the fact Jimmy made a cash payment of twelve thousand dollars for a used van. His bank statements showed no record of a deposit or a withdrawal for twelve thousand dollars, this included both his business account and his personal account.

Sometimes that's the way it is with cash, Kate thought, it just appears, but on the heels of a high-profile robbery, I don't think so. 'Any good investigator would dig into this a little deeper was Kate's last thought.

That evening Kate and Sonny compared notes and told each other of their findings. What they had wasn't much but you have to keep digging, that's the way it is in the investigating business, keep digging, and they both knew it.

Carman Fish and Charmain Green drove up to San Francisco on a day off from work. The main purpose of the drive was to open a factious bank account, but it was also a relaxing getaway day.

Two days after their return to San St. Rosalina, Carman had two million dollars wired from the Swiss bank account to the account in San Francisco. On that same day, Cameron Blue's bank account in Bellevue, Washington, was fatten by over a half million dollars.

Carman made two additional trips to the Bay Area, and money was moved to different places by different means at different times. By early February, each thief had received over five hundred thousand dollars in payoffs, except Roxanne Rodriquez and Cameron Blue.

Roxanne Rodriquez's bank account was already fat due of her marriage to the Brazilian coffee Barron. One day on a quiet afternoon over lunch, Roxy tells Carman to give her share of the money to Cameron.

"I don't need the money, Carman, I don't want the money, it was never about the money and if I ever do need money I'll look you up."

"Cameron needs over three hundred thousand dollars just for the operation, and then there is recovery time. There is the possibility of complications setting in; I don't want him to be worried over finances. Give him my share of the money and tell him to keep the change." "I love Cameron, I think he is one of the greatest persons I've met, and I want to do my part to make sure all goes well for him, at least financially. He's been waiting a long time for this."

"Yes, I hear you, Roxy, I will see to it that your wish is carried out. I agree with you, Cameron is a great guy, and he is going to need extra help. I'll make sure he gets your share of the money and anything else he needs."

"What are you and Charmain going to do after Florida?"

"We're going to spend a little time in Florida, maybe two or three weeks, nothing serious visiting family and friends, no jobs or anything like that. Then it's off to Iowa for more of the same. I've always wanted to live in South Africa, maybe learn how to surf, enjoy the beaches, the sunshine, eat seafood, we'll see."

"I know one thing for sure; we'll be by the ocean."

"I hear you; the ocean is a big part of my life as well. Just seeing the sea, hearing the sound of the waves and smelling the freshness of the salt air can make a big difference in a person's life."

"A steady diet of fresh seafood definitely beats farmed cows and cooped chickens. We've been lucky, Carman, we could have been born in North Texas, Wyoming, or Idaho and missed out on this ocean life. I wouldn't trade it for anything."

"We must always stay in touch."